The Body Cooperative

The Body Cooperative

*Essential Elements of
Human Health—And How to
Make Them Work for You*

DR. SAM SLATTERY

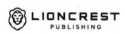

Hardcover ISBN: 978-1-5445-3296-7
Paperback ISBN: 978-1-5445-3297-4
Ebook ISBN: 978-1-5445-3298-1

To the many people who brought me to this place and those who I hope will benefit in some way from its contents.

CONTENTS

Introduction ix

PART I
Beginning Your Journey 1

    CHAPTER 1
    Making a Plan .3

    CHAPTER 2
    Understanding the Science 13

PART II
The Five Elements 43

    CHAPTER 3
    Decoding Diet 45

    CHAPTER 4
    Essential Exercise 83

    CHAPTER 5
    Get Some Sleep 103

    CHAPTER 6
    It's All about Me-Time 123

    CHAPTER 7
    Manage That Stress 133

PART III

Executing on Your Plan. 155

CHAPTER 8

Barriers to Change. 157

CHAPTER 9

Putting It All Together. 185

Conclusion 195

Recommended Reading. 205

Acknowledgments 207

About the Author 211

INTRODUCTION

I am a doctor—and I am here to tell you *not* to go to doctors for health advice.

Is this a controversial statement? Perhaps…but it shouldn't be.

Most doctors only learn how to fix sickness. They are trained in one style, and many are narrow-minded in their views. In many countries, medical doctors have highjacked the healing space when, in reality, most have almost no knowledge about how to be healthy. Nutrition is not even a class taught in many medical schools!

Of course, I'm making a sweeping generalization, but in all honesty, the average doctor gets about two hours of training in nutrition and virtually none in exercise or sleep. They know little about the skills required to reflect on mental and physical health. Their experience of stress management is often only that of managing their own stress. But most importantly, they have a poor understanding of the connections between the mind and the body. They see their patients as being made up of individual systems and suffering from isolated diseases—and those doctors fail to recognize the person as a whole. This is a fundamental flaw in medical thinking and treatment.

My late mother used to say, "A good doctor's job is to provide health advice to people so that they can continue to enjoy the things they love without killing themselves any sooner than necessary."

With those words, she captured so many important concepts that we have forgotten. We are individuals and indeed unique. There is no average human. Each of us has our own makeup, both physically and emotionally. Each of us has our own needs in terms of enjoying the things that we love.

In the past, a medical doctor's role was to "cure rarely, relieve suffering often, and comfort always." Today it is "cure always (impossible), relieve suffering if you have time, and ask others to provide comfort and compassion."

The old way was powerful medicine because it recognized the importance of the person, and it worked. Health is about the well-being of a whole individual, not just the absence of sickness and disease. Furthermore, as you will discover, you cannot separate the person and their mind from their physical health.

That's why this book is different.

Who Am I?

But who am I? And why should you listen to me? After all, I told you that I, too, am a doctor, right?

Yes, I'm a doctor. But I'm not your typical doctor. First, I treat *people*, not diseases, which makes me a bit of a dinosaur in modern medical circles. Second, I understand my role in individuals' lives. The word *doctor* comes from the Latin *docere*, to teach. As a physician, my job is to educate, advise, and assist. It is not my role to be your mother or other authority and tell you what to do. It's your life, and how you live it is your choice. But I can educate and empower you with knowledge that enables you to make decisions based on sound information and facts. My job is to be up to date and effectively share that knowledge with you in terms that you can understand.

Recognizing that I am not the source of all the answers, I keep an open mind, working with patients as partners. They are a significant source of my experience and knowledge as a physician.

I have spent forty years in the trenches dealing with every type of sickness. During that time, I became increasingly frustrated by the endless failures. Many of my patients may have improved, but they did not become well. I often felt that I was simply handing out medication, which made their numbers look better, but it was often just Band-Aid medicine. In partnership, we were just papering over the cracks.

My big wake-up call came when I was forty-five years old. I became sick, and not one doctor could help me.

Ill, overwhelmed, and frightened, it dawned on me that I was a patient with a seemingly incurable disease. I was chronically fatigued, had constant stomach pain, and depressed. My mind was often foggy and unclear. I had strange bowel movements, and my joints felt like they were those of an old man. I struggled to balance my work and family commitments. Worst of all was the constant pain from the ulcers lining my entire mouth. I was exhausted, with no help in sight and nowhere to go.

Oh, sure, I had medical help. I had a cardiologist for my abnormal heart rhythms and a rheumatologist for the joint pain that left me crippled every morning. I had a gastroenterologist because my guts felt like they were on fire all the time, an internal medicine specialist, and a GP.

Five different doctors, not counting me—and none of them could figure out why I was in unrelenting pain with these debilitating symptoms.

I had blood tests. Then a cardiac stress test with an echocardiogram. They put cameras into both ends of my guts. (I'll come back to that fun test later because, as it happens, it turned out to be the clue that helped me unravel the problem.) The biopsies were all normal, so it was clear I did not have celiac disease or apparently any other "real" illness.

But all those educated colleagues could not fix me. They told me that I was stressed out and "neurotic"—which was partly correct. But implying that someone is neurotic is the dumping ground of the diagnostically destitute and the wilderness for their patients, which is not very helpful if you *are* the patient.

I was sick, and nobody knew what to do except make me feel guilty, which only made me feel worse. Somehow it was my fault.

I felt frightened and alone.

Diagnosing Myself (With a Little Help!)

In the back of my mind, my illness seemed to be related to food. Food became the enemy, and I was afraid to eat.

Then a specialist ordered yet another round of tests—including my second colonoscopy in five years. I was still experiencing the same symptoms, but my colonoscopy and endoscopy were reported as normal; "just a bit of very mild inflammation," I was told. (Here lay the clue.)

Yet again, I went home without a diagnosis from the doctors. I was so frustrated about having to do these invasive tests without getting any answers—and without ever feeling any better!

But something had changed. After my colonoscopy bowel prep, I felt better. I thought about this for a couple of days, and then the penny dropped. The last time I felt like this was after my last colonoscopy and bowel prep. I thought, *Maybe something was poisoning me in my bowel, and when I flushed it out, I got better!*

Then, as life goes, I saw a patient—a high school teacher—who had previously told me to stop eating wheat. This was in 2009, when not much was yet known about wheat intolerance. In my mind, it was the latest fad diagnosis and not for me—a clever, balanced, and educated doctor!

But I didn't have any better theories, so I gave it a try and went wheat-free. We would now call this going "gluten-free" because gluten is the cause of celiac disease, and doctors recognize the word. It is indeed the protein in wheat that in part causes the problems associated with digestive health and gut inflammation, but that is not the whole wheat story. Hence, wheat-free is the correct term.

Much to my surprise and everyone else's, I got better—and quickly, too. In a matter of a few days, I noticed a difference, and within a couple of weeks, I was 80 percent of the way back to my previously healthier self.

I started to experiment with changing other things in my diet, and no longer as much of a surprise, everything got even better. I discovered something else. I liked feeling well and being full of energy. I enjoyed the new me a lot.

So at age forty-five, I went back to school to learn what medical school had never taught me: how to be healthy.

What I learned was unexpected, but in hindsight obvious. I, like my doctors, had been focusing on my symptoms and gut behaviors, entirely missing a fundamental question: why had this happened to me? Not to just my gut and my joints—*me*, the whole person. The answer was a highly stressful life with a poor diet, minimal exercise, and too much alcohol. I had walked myself into ill health with my lifestyle. Ultimately, I had sensitized my gut to wheat and corn, among other things, and created an entire body that was out of balance, very inflamed, and extremely sick.

As my knowledge grew, I came to understand that behind this layer was another—something more complex and difficult to address—something that began many years before I got sick, before I was even in charge of my own lifestyle.

I, like so many, had a childhood that was challenging and difficult. On the face of it, all should have been well. My parents were educated professionals. We had a nice home and a good education at fine schools. But behind this façade, all was not so well. (I could write a book about this part of my life, but that's for another time.)

The trauma of being separated from my parents at the age of seven. The unique challenges and indeed horrors of Jesuit boarding school, and the nightmare of being alone without help. The events that left deep scars. All this against other traumas, unhappy parents, and their divorce when I was twelve, leading to the next being "sent away" to another boarding school.

Suffice to say that I can now, from a place of experience and knowledge, understand how my body was primed by my childhood for the meltdown that was to come. We will explore this important aspect of becoming unwell later in the book.

This is not a "poor me" account. Far from it. It was in fact critical to who I am and perhaps what I do. I learned to survive, and it made me tough, though the scars took a long time to heal. Indeed, some never will. But it is also a time that I now consider a blessing because I gained something. It gave me empathy for others because I learned that we all suffer in some way, and to be the best you is to recognize this truth and strive to alleviate suffering in others if you can. Even those who did me harm were themselves the product of damaging childhoods.

My Journey to Healthy Living

Once I recognized the causes and had the light-bulb moment that illness was a full-body event, I started the journey that I still pursue to this day. My mission involved learning how our bodies—and, equally importantly, our minds and brains—actually work.

I studied nutrition, exercise, sleep, mindfulness, and meditation. I discovered the science that explains why who we are is dictated to a great extent by what life throws at us. I learned how poor diet leads to a distressed colony of bacteria inside our gut and the inflammation that this derangement causes in the wall of the intestine, along with the molecular science behind leaky guts. I discovered how this inflammation leads to an unbalanced *neuro-immune system*, and in turn an inflamed and distressed, foggy brain, along with a weakened body. How this alteration of the neuro-immune system causes obscure and seemingly separate symptoms, like palpitations and actual abnormal heart rhythms, along with very real and well-documented illnesses like Parkinson's disease, eczema, diabetes, and cancer.

I enhanced my psychological knowledge and skills, coming to understand why we continue to partake in habits that we know hurt us and why so many of us fail to stick with life choices that we all recognize will make us feel well. I discovered that our childhood background and storyline, and indeed even our mother's health and experiences before and during pregnancy, predict our own physical and mental health life story.

I examined biochemistry at a level never taught in medical school. I listened to numerous cutting-edge podcasts, read health and nutrition blogs, and reviewed thousands of leading papers on a wide range of basic science and medical topics.

Finally, and most important of all, I studied how the gut works. I gained a master's degree in gastroenterology and nutrition from London University. This education in neuro-immunology of the gut underpinned my ongoing quest to understand its central role in human health and illness.

I started to apply my new and ever-expanding health knowledge to myself and my patients. We found that when we changed a few simple things, we began to heal and feel better.

So why trust me?

xvi • The Body Cooperative

I'll tell you straight up: because I have successfully helped hundreds of people make the same journey, whether from sickness to health or from already-mostly-healthy to even-*healthier*.

And, with some of the common-sense information in this book, *you* can begin your journey to improved health and start to feel better, too!

This Book Is for *You*

By this point, you might still be wondering, *Is this book really for me?*

If you are wondering if this book is for you, the short answer is yes.

Well, let me ask you:

- Do you want to try to stay healthy for your whole life? (Of course you do.)

- Are you feeling run down, fatigued, overweight, and generally unhappy with your current state of health? (I'm going to guess that you think life could be better.)

- Are you worried about the future, aging, and all its worrisome medical bills? (You should be.)

- Do you feel your clothes are way too snug, or have you lost sight of your toes when you look down? (Hmmmm.)

- Are your intimate relationships and sex life struggling and un-fulfilling? (Likely.)

- Do you wonder why you often drag yourself through the day? (Another coffee, please!)

- Are you envious of those who seem to enjoy eternal youth? (How do they stay so young?)

- Are you frustrated by the endless stream of contradictory health and wellness advice? (What's the difference anyway?)

- Are you tired of hearing or reading about yet another fad diet, the latest fitness craze, or supplements that will save you? (Not today, Facebook!)

- Do you want to have a basic understanding of yourself and how you work inside, both mind and body? (It's not so complicated.)

- Most importantly, especially for those of you who are struggling from both physical and mental health challenges, do you want to *feel better*? (I know you do.)

If you answered "yes, please!" to any of these questions…you're in the right place.

Additionally, if you have IBS, chronic pain, palpitations, chronic anxiety, or long-term mental health challenges—or have been labeled as having an illness without a known cause or explanation—this book is also for you. Contrary to popular medical belief, it's not all in your head. You are not being neurotic or difficult; you have a very real medical condition. As you move through the book, you are going to learn how to cope with your problem, how to reduce your symptoms—and possibly remove them completely. You will come to understand the importance of mental health.

xviii • *The Body Cooperative*

It is entirely possible to improve your life, whether you already suffer from a health challenge and want to feel better, or you desire to prevent future health problems so that you can continue living your best life and enjoy the things you love. Although it sounds obvious, the best solution is to be as healthy as possible, which is not necessarily the complete absence of disease or illness.

This book is intended for anyone who wants a simple but definitive and comprehensive guide to achieving better health. If you are already a "biohacker" who listens to leading health podcasts and avidly reads cutting-edge health blogs, then this book might be short of fine detail for you. (However, as it provides a skeleton for *anyone* to organize, formalize, and rationalize their thoughts…you'll probably find that you get something quite useful out of it!)

Understanding how the body works is complicated if you want to get down into the nitty-gritty. But in spite of all the confusing detail, being healthy is actually easy. The body knows how to run itself, and indeed heal, if you give it a chance.

And this book is a common-sense guide to teach you how to do exactly that.

Dispelling Common Myths and Misconceptions

Before we get into *how* to be healthy, I first want to dispel some common myths and misconceptions.

Myth #1: You need to see a doctor to be healthy. No! Most doctors have minimal or no training in health; most of us are educated only in managing sickness. Doctors are trained to "fix" people when they are "broken," usually through the use of medicines or surgery. Why? That's what they know. Worse, doctors are increasingly specialized, with the inevitable result that they do not understand or see the whole person and the big picture, which is so critical to health.

Myth #2: Lifespan has increased. Not much, perhaps ten years. True, life *expectancy*—or the likelihood of reaching your *lifespan*—has increased. Infant mortality has dropped, manual work is much safer, and improvements in sanitation, vaccines, and housing have led to a massive decrease in infectious diseases, so more children reach old age. This raises life- expectancy figures.

The median lifespan, however, for healthy, appropriately nourished humans has remained around seventy to eighty years of age for more than 2,000 years. (There are good records from ancient Greece, Egypt, and Rome recognizing centenarians!) You can assume that a lifespan somewhere between eighty to ninety years is realistic. (You might be surprised to discover that traditional people like the Hazda hunter-gatherers, with no access to modern anything, if they survive childhood, typically reach these ages in excellent health.) Plan accordingly.

Myth #3: Increased life expectancy is due to doctors. Nope. The number-one reason for the increased life expectancy, in our crowded urbanized world, as we just discussed, is improved sanitation. The second reason is improved living conditions, and the third is decreased infections—which is primarily due to reasons one and two, along with vaccines. These are public health initiatives.

Additionally, after the 1980s, the fatality rate of heart attacks fell by 50 percent in the US. Most of this was due to lifestyle changes in the population, including decreased smoking rates. Even where there was medical intervention, 50 percent of the reduction was still due to supervised lifestyle changes, not medication. Rates would have fallen further, but the massive increase in obesity and diabetes reversed the gains. Heart disease was rare before the 1900s!

A scary but true, sobering fact: life expectancy is currently falling in both the US and indeed the UK. Current lifestyles and our toxic environment are now reversing the gains of the last few decades.

Myth #4: Aging means you become ill. Not true. Advancing age does not mean your joints naturally fail and your internal organs predictably wear out. These events should occur at the very end of your life, not start at age thirty. Most of us become ill because we don't look after our body and our mind—but that's not a criticism. How can you be successful if you don't know what to do? We age prematurely and suffer due to excess inflammation caused by our modern lifestyles.

Myth #5: Becoming unwell, having heart disease, developing arthritis, and getting cancer are a matter of your genes. Nothing could be further from the truth. In fact, only perhaps 4 percent to 8 percent of these conditions can be attributed to your inherited genetic code. The rest is actually a matter of environment, your childhood, and your chosen lifestyle. In other words, the way we live influences the expression of our genetic code: a process known as epigenetics.

Myth #6: Positive visualization helps us change. No again; the evidence does not support this. Indeed, it's quite the opposite. It can set you up for failure, and failure is not good for you.

Myth #7: Being healthy is expensive. Not necessarily. Being *unhealthy* is expensive—think of the costs of doctors' bills, insurance, and medications. Healthy choices, on the other hand—such as exercise, sleep, Me-Time, and stress management (more on these in a moment!)—are mostly free. And even those that are not free—food, for example—can be inexpensive if you know what to buy. Vegetables are a very good example of this.

Myth #8: Being healthy is time consuming. Again, not true. If you think living a healthy lifestyle takes too much time, consider what happens when you lose your health: time off work, doctors' visits, hospital stays…you get the picture.

Myth #9: Being healthy means no fun. Far from it! Good health empowers you to live life to the fullest in every sense of the word—well into your seventies and beyond in good condition.

Myth #10: I need self-discipline. No, you don't. You just need to let go of fear and start making one small step or change. Stop overthinking and just do something. Doing is the key!

Bonus Myth:
Being Overweight Does Not Matter

Sorry. I know this is hurtful to many, but weight does matter. It's just a fact. I know that losing it is challenging and that many need help, but you need to do it on so many levels. We should all strive to find our personal body type and genetically programmed weight. For most of us, that's much less than we weigh today.

The Five Key Elements to Better Health

Now let's look at the five simple elements that make up the magic formula to better health.

Diet: We've all heard it: you are what you eat! It's true, and we now understand why. Hidden inside your intestines is a colony of bacteria that have a significant influence on how your body and mind operate. Eat the wrong types of food and you end up with an inflammatory colony that prematurely ages your body, contributes to you being overweight, and makes you miserable. Eat the right food, however, and you will build a healthy ecosystem of microorganisms that does precisely the opposite by balancing the neuro-immune system in the gut wall.

Exercise: We are a biodynamic machine made of moving parts, and to keep those parts in good working order, we need to move. There's no escaping this simple truth—but that doesn't mean you have to become a gym rat, yoga junky, or marathon runner. Simply recognize the importance of movement and get some daily exercise in whatever form you *enjoy*.

Sleep: This is an incredibly complex process, and one that is crucial for health. Sleep is when your body and brain clean house. They repair damage and reset systems back to their baseline. During this time, the brain washes away debris from the day's work; your intestine cleans itself; and the liver flushes out the toxins built up during the previous sixteen hours. This is one of the most essential elements, and you don't have to do anything but go to bed!

Me-Time: This is time you spend being with yourself to reflect upon how you are doing physically, mentally, and emotionally. If you don't pay attention to yourself, how can you know if the adjustments you are making are harmful or beneficial? This increased self-reflection will also lead to improved self-awareness and mindfulness.

Stress Management: Life is stressful. That's a fact, and there is no escaping it. In itself, stress may not be harmful. (Indeed, it can be beneficial, as it can motivate us.) It is the strain produced by stress that is damaging to us. But strain can be managed. The first four elements—eating a nutritious diet, engaging in physical activity, developing healthy sleep habits, and practicing regular Me-Time—all provide a firm foundation for stress and strain management.

None of these elements are secret, new, or clever. I'm sure it's nothing that you have not heard before. All I have done is put them into one book and explained why they are important and how they are linked.

In fact, as I was writing this book, I worried that people would say, "This is all just common sense."

But that's the point, isn't it? It *is* just common sense, but we need to put it all together, and then we need to *do* something. No amount of thinking, visualizing, wishing, and praying will change anything. You have to be a doer to change the way you think and feel.

An Overview of Your Journey

The journey to better health is just that: a journey. Journeys are made up of a series of small steps. As long as you're heading in the right direction, each step will take you closer to your goal.

Think of this book as your guide through that journey. Each chapter highlights one major element and helps define the stages along the way.

Of course, if you don't start the journey, you're never going to reach your new destination!

To make your journey easier, I have divided the book into three parts:

- Part I is the beginning of your journey. In it, you will learn to make a plan, as well as some foundational, scientific concepts that will become your tools moving forward.

- Part II is the main part of your journey, wherein we will discuss each of the Five Elements in greater detail.

- Part III may just be the most difficult portion of your journey. In it, you will execute on the plan created in Part I. To do so, however, you will first have to overcome your barriers to change. Finally, all the components of your plan can come together so that improved health can be yours!

At the end of each chapter, you will find your "To-Do List"—a page that includes important takeaways from the chapter you've just read, as well as specific steps preparing you to tackle the next element. Do the things on that To-Do List, and you will find that your health improves.

And that's it! This journey will transform your life. Best of all, it is simple, inexpensive, and within everyone's reach.

Perhaps you are thinking, *Easier said than done*. Well, nothing worth doing is ever completely free of some effort.

When you pick up a book, you are confronted with pages of writing—and this book is no exception. Indeed, it is longer than the average book today, which can be off-putting for even the most avid reader. Why? Because most of us are busy and don't have the time for long, detailed reading. You want information in the most straightforward format possible.

I have constructed the book in such a way that you can choose how you want to use it. You can take a quick overview, read some detailed passages, or read it all. Although all of the information is related, you can read the chapters in any order you wish. If you want to get the most out of your journey, don't neglect any of the Five Elements! All are critical components to being healthy. And after you've read a chapter, use your To-Do List as a reminder of what you've read—and what comes next.

I know it's all a bit heavy, and I have done my best to lighten up the style, but I promise that everything you read is carefully researched and will be thought provoking. Some of what you are about to learn is cutting-edge knowledge. You will literally be one of the earliest to ride this new wave of understanding of how the body works.

Remember, all adventures begin with a single step. Most of us don't start because we feel overwhelmed by the seemingly complicated and challenging task ahead. But you deserve congratulations because you've already taken that first step: you picked up this book. Allow me to be your guide, and let's continue the journey together so you can begin to enjoy the benefits of a clear and simple plan for living well. The ultimate goal? The motivation to make the effort to extend your *healthspan* (the period of your life spent in good health) as close to your lifespan (the time you live) as possible—and to extend your lifespan as close to, or even beyond, current life expectancy.

Are you ready to clarify your mind, discover your body, and improve your health, all while making your life so much more fulfilling? Keep reading.

PART I

BEGINNING YOUR JOURNEY

. . . .

CHAPTER 1

MAKING A PLAN

. . . .

I tried to give up smoking for twenty-five years. I read books. I tried hypnosis and acupuncture. I meditated and visualized myself as a nonsmoker, thinking about all the money I would save. I imagined myself with lung cancer (which just made me anxious and smoke more). I tried positive affirmation, applied logical thought—heck, even *illogical* thought. I tried everything (at least I thought I had), but I was never successful for long. At the end of all those efforts, I was consuming forty cigarettes per day!

Then one day the light went on. I stopped thinking about how to quit, and I did something. I made the decision that I really did want to stop, and then I made a plan. I wrote it down, and then I just *did it*—I followed the plan. Within two weeks I was a nonsmoker. I don't mean I didn't smoke; I mean I was a nonsmoker: I didn't *feel* like a smoker; I didn't *think* like a smoker; and most important of all...*I didn't smoke.* That was in 2001, and even now, decades later, I still don't smoke.

My experience with alcohol was different. Unlike stopping cigarettes, which I did quickly and cleanly, my move away from anything but infrequent drinks was more gradual.

As is the case with many of us, I was never a good drinker, and although I was a happy person when I enjoyed too much, I realized it wasn't me. I hated hangovers, even the very mild ones resulting after two drinks. I wanted to stop.

I started drinking less, and when I did, I felt better. So I concentrated on how good it was to feel well in the morning. As time went by, I realized that I had started to make an active decision between having a drink and feeling a bit off the next day, or having no alcohol and feeling great and sharp in the morning—and the rest of the day, for that matter. I had chosen feeling great. The result was that I stopped drinking on a regular basis, and I've never regretted it.

Nobody told me that I should not drink. No one said it was bad for my health. But because I began to pay attention to what happened when I drank, I made some new choices. My change came about because I was mindful and aware.

Changing my diet was different yet again. In this case, there was no choice. I had, like so many others, become overweight and sick. I now understand that a poor diet coupled with immense amounts of stress caused my gut to "melt down," with the consequence that I developed IBS of the worst kind. My entire health failed, as I shared with you in the Introduction of this book.

Although an extremely challenging part of my life, it was in hindsight a blessing. It started me on the journey that not only regained my health but led me to being healthier than I had ever been. It also allowed me to assist many other people from a place of knowledge and experience.

Plan for Success

The product of my journey to better health is an intimate understanding of how the process of change works.

If you want to be healthy, you also have to understand how health happens. Knowledge is power because it enables you to make your own decisions—and it is only when you have decided to change that you can actually make that change. Let me reassure you, it's not so complex that you cannot follow. Anyone can learn how the process works.

Change occurs in a stepwise manner.

The first step is called *pre-contemplation.* This is the recognition that you need to make adjustments to your life. This is a mulling-over process that can take weeks and months, possibly years. It's that "I need to do something" feeling.

The next is the process of *contemplation.* This is the stage when you actively start thinking about how to modify parts of your life. It's when you begin to consider the details.

Then we start planning the actual steps: the *preparation* phase. We do research, figure out which gym to join or diet we think might be the best. We use friends, books like this one, pamphlets, and TV adverts to decide what we are going to do.

Next comes *action.* We try to carry out the plan and change how we behave.

If we persist, we then enter the *consolidation* phase. We continue the new behavior. If we do so for long enough to recognize the benefits, it can become a habit.

However, this is the most difficult and challenging part of the process. Often we do not carry on long enough, or something drags us back to the old ways. We *relapse.* This is the critical issue when it comes to failure to change. We need to come up with a solution to address this event—and, in reality, it's very simple.

The good news is that there is a way to create lasting change in your life. It's called "Make a Plan." Yes, it is that straightforward.

Think about it. What do all successful people have in common? Simple, a plan.

"Maybe they're just lucky," you may say. To that I respond, "There is no such thing as luck. Good fortune is created by planning and adaptability. The solution to any problem is to develop a plan and then try it."

To be successful, you need to make a plan to specifically address the challenges that arise in the *action* and *consolidation* phases to prevent *relapse*. Even if you do relapse, have a plan to minimize the effect on your final goal. If you do this, then you can and most likely will succeed. If you do not, then it's just like the old adage says: fail to plan, plan to fail.

How to Make a Plan

Obvious as it may seem, the first step to having a plan is to make one. It never fails to amaze me how often people will have great ideas, with appropriate aspirations and goals…but no detailed plan. Little wonder so many are unsuccessful in their quest for a different life.

First ask yourself, "What am I trying to achieve?"

My guess is that you want to be healthier; otherwise, you would not have picked up this book. Other guesses would be that you want to be a different shape, fitter, happier, or, more importantly, more content.

So grab your notebook or a piece of paper and let's start.

I want you to make five headings, one for each of the Five Elements. (I know you haven't yet read those chapters, but there is an overview of each in the Introduction, and none of these elements should be unfamiliar to you. As you read each chapter, you can update your plan, and we'll take a look at it again in Chapter 9.)

Make sure there is some space beneath each heading. (I like to use a page for each.) Now, under each element, write down your *goal* for that element.

For example, under the heading Diet, you might choose to write "I want to stop eating sugar." Under Exercise, write something like "I want to be able to walk two flights of stairs at work without being short of breath." (Your goals don't have to be too difficult. Be realistic.)

Next, under each goal, you will write your *motivation* for achieving that goal. These are your own reasons for wanting to change things. They need to be personal and deeply held feelings at an emotional level.

For example, under "I want to stop eating sugar," you might write reasons such as "I want to lose weight because I'm embarrassed." It does not matter how silly the reason feels. It's yours, and it's private, but it must be deeply felt. This is critical because if you don't have a deeply felt motivating reason, you will fail. In short, you must *want* to change rather than think you *need* to. There is a difference.

Once you've come up with motivating reasons for each goal under each element, you are going to write your plan. This gets a bit more challenging because plans have steps and parts to them. You need to get into the details here.

First, write out the steps you are going to take to achieve your goals. (Do this for each of your five headings.)

For example, the Diet heading might now look something like this:

- Diet

    • **Goal:** I want to stop eating sugar.

    • **Motivation:** I want to lose weight because I'm embarrassed.

    • **Steps:**

        ▪ Remove all sugar from the house.

        ▪ Stop buying sugar and all sugary drinks, such as juice and sodas.

- Read all food labels before buying and see how much sugar is in the product.

- Have an excuse when friends or family offer me foods containing sugar.

- Have non-sugary foods available for when I am craving sugar.

Finally, and most important, you have to follow your plan.

It really is that simple. But let's look at a couple of guidelines to help you become successful.

Be Realistic

As you start your journey, a small word of caution: let's be realistic.

Genetics do play a role. Look at your family. There are traits that lifestyle will not overcome, such as the basic design and build of your body or your height, for example. But don't get too hung up on your family health history. Your own mental attitude and lifestyle is the significant predictor of your health destiny.

In my own journey, I never lost sight of certain truths. It was going to take a lot of gym time to turn me into a muscular man—in fact, way more time than my life had available. I started as Mr. "Puniverse," not Mr. Universe, and several years in, I can still be best described as Mr. Puniverse-Plus! I keep my aspirations real. I have never envisioned having a six-pack or making the front cover of *GQ*. That way, I am never disappointed.

As you write down your goals, make sure they are realistic and achievable. Start with easy-to-reach targets that include the endpoint and the timeline. For example, you might choose a reasonable target of losing five pounds in two months—but not twenty pounds in one month! Shoot for five minutes of exercise per day, not a marathon next month. Decide to bring bedtime forward fifteen minutes, not an entire hour.

Remember, we are looking for victories, not failures. So set yourself up for success and make sure to celebrate those victories. But not with a tub of ice cream! A scoop, perhaps? Moderation in all things.

Embrace the New You

How you approach your plan—and the inevitable challenges that will arise—is the key to long-term success in making lifestyle changes.

Your mindset and actions shape who you are. The way you choose to think about things, and the way you express those thoughts, will influence how you feel and behave. It is critical that you understand this most important psychological fact: your thoughts create your reality. We live by the series of stories we construct in our minds.

Here are two very different and potential internal dialogues after successfully giving up sugar for a week.

I don't know why I gave up sugar. I really miss the sugar in my coffee every morning. Life is no fun. Worse, yesterday I could not eat any of that cake and donuts that Jennifer brought to the office. Everybody else was enjoying theirs. I felt so left out. This isn't going to work. This is too difficult. I'm not happy about the change. I'm miserable.

Versus:

Wow, success. I managed to go a whole week without sugar. The first couple of days were a bit challenging—very hard, actually—but then I decided to feel good about it and just take it a day at a time. At the beginning it was odd and difficult, but I kept reminding myself that it was going to be worth it. I even managed to avoid the cake and donuts Jennifer brought to the office yesterday. (I stuck to the steps in my plan to deal with this challenge.) That made me feel really good because I was in control. And I have to admit I do feel better. I'm glad that I had a go at this. I am so encouraged to carry on.

Reading those two paragraphs, how do you feel? Same scenario, but very different attitudes, thoughts, and words. This is how your own brain works. It has a direct influence on your personal reality and thus your chance of achieving improved health.

How you feel motivates you to continue. Take every small success as a significant step forward. It's challenging to keep going if you feel negative about what you are doing. But it becomes easier to carry on when you focus on the gains, not the losses.

One of my old psychology teachers used to say, "Tell patients to clean up their language." He was correct. You have to be mindful of what you think and say. When you hear yourself becoming negative, stop it. Change the dialogue to a positive one. Express it in words and, better still, write it down. You'll be surprised to find that how you feel will begin to change.

Your To-Do List

Your to-do list consists of the four process phases that you will work through when you want to make a change in your life.

PRE-CONTEMPLATION

1. Take stock of your life. Make a list of what you want to change.

2. Recognize *why* you want to change.

CONTEMPLATION

1. Make a decision that you are going to change and how. The Goal(s).

PREPARATION

1. Make a commitment to keeping a simple notebook. *Write* in your book what your goals are and why you want to hit that goal. Your motivations need to be real and deeply personal. This is crucial.

2. Then think about a plan. How are you going to get there?

3. Finally, ask yourself, "Are my goals realistic?"

4. Prepare a plan to specifically deal with the consolidation phase. This is one of the key points in the process. This is where it will go wrong if you don't have specific plans for the challenges that will naturally arise.

5. Make sure that you write out each step of the plan.

ACTION AND CONSOLIDATION

1. Carry out the plan(s) for a sufficiently long enough period to experience the benefits—at least three months, but six is even better.

Keep it simple. If it's too complicated, you will struggle to follow it. You should be able to do all of the above over a cup coffee—well perhaps two (no sugar).

Remember, psychology teaches us that change occurs in a stepwise fashion over a period of time. Be patient, but keep moving forward. As you succeed to reach your first goal for any element, if you want, set a new one and just repeat the process.

And now you're on your way!

You've taken a huge step by making a plan to change, but this is only the first step in your journey. There's more to learn before you can fully enact your plan. Your next step is to grasp some foundational scientific concepts about what's happening inside you and what could happen if you *don't* make some of these changes. Chapter 2 will provide sufficient information to help you understand how the body works. But don't panic; it's not rocket science!

CHAPTER 2

UNDERSTANDING
THE SCIENCE
. . . .

You are not really a human as you understand it—you are, both numerically and genetically, at best only 30 percent human! Shocked? Read on.

Your body is a large ecosystem: a meta-organism made up of many different cells, both human and non-human. This astonishing mix works in an integrated and cooperative manner to create us, *Homo sapiens*.

We are like a tropical rainforest, ancient woodland, or coral reef where all the different species of plants and animal or fish life are interdependent, requiring each other to maintain a healthy whole. We represent the pinnacle of millions of years of evolution on this planet, a complex ecosystem that is mobile and can manipulate its own fate.

Think of individual cell types as different species of animals and organs as unique habitats. This is not an idle analogy; your different cell types and your non-human partners are as different as a whale might be from a chimpanzee, a tree from a fern, or a forest from a lake.

Our skin is like the desert, dry and harsh, but within this desert are oases—places like our armpits and groins that are moist and have unique ecosystems. Our back is different from our front; our palms are different from the soles of our feet. Our nose has a different colony from our mouth, and our intestines provide the richest environment of all—indeed, one of the most diverse and complex bacterial ecosystems on Earth. This is exactly like different ecosystems on our planet. Totally different animals live in the desert as compared to a forest or a river. There are also vertical habitats, just like in a rainforest, where the animals and birds living in the tops of trees are completely different from those living on the forest floor.

The Science Inside You

The workings of the body are as complex as the universe. The challenge of unraveling the millions of variables makes studying the human body an infinitely complicated task. But in spite of a significant lack of detail, we have worked out a general picture. So why, you might ask, is there so much conflicting advice about how to be healthy and well?

Part of the problem is the way that science works. It tends to be compartmentalized. Different scientific disciplines work in isolation with limited cross-communication and sharing of ideas between specialties. So, as we become increasingly sophisticated in investigating the details, we have lost the ability to see the forest for the trees. Individuals present the views of their area of knowledge but struggle to place them into a larger picture. The disappearance of generalists like myself who stitch together the detailed pieces of knowledge created by specialist and sub-specialist researchers is an ever-increasing problem. It leads to distorted and fragmented advice based on snippets of information rather than the whole.

Other challenges include various biases, a concept that we will explore later, and funding, which tends to unbalance research.

Sadly, quite a lot of what you have been told is at best out of date, and a great deal is actually wrong.

Before you can relearn the best ways to become healthier, we must first establish some essential baseline knowledge about the workings of your body.

In this chapter, you will discover that you need to develop balanced nervous and immune systems (which, as you will see, are the housekeepers of our bodies), endocrine system, and gut, which contains your microbiome. The key threat to the body and your well-being is *inflammation* caused by an imbalance in these systems.

We will examine the critical but ignored mind-body connection, including the scientific disciplines of *psychoneuroimmunology* and the closely related subject of *psychoneuroendocrinology*. These connections explain how what you think and feel, along with the environment you live in, have a profound influence on your health.

It is through an appreciation of these systems that you will find a better way to live your life—not because the doctor told you to do something, but because you will understand what drives your body and how you can fix it. Your goal: a healthy, and hopefully *long*, life.

The Neuro-Immune System

Traditionally, we have divided the study of the human body into artificial compartments—the nervous system, cardiovascular system, digestive system, immune system—as if they exist in isolation. This limited view can create an unrealistic understanding.

The body is not made up of individual systems or parts. Indeed, it is quite the opposite. It is composed of groups of specialist cells that are best understood as an integrated and intricate ecosystem established on cooperative behavior. This structure requires sophisticated communication and negotiating skills between cells based on a complex language and an ability to keep the peace.

At the heart of the human body is the *neuro-immune system*: a group of cells that have coevolved to evaluate the internal and external environment and then share this information with all other cells.

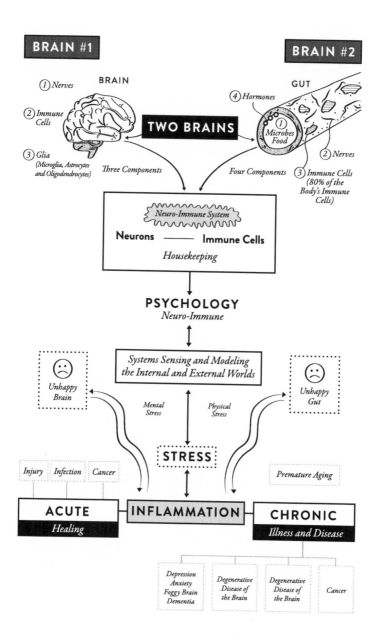

This system, made up of two specialist branches, is the "backbone" of the human body. It is the system that allows all other cells in the body to survive and function in a safe and "friendly" environment. It is similar to the structure of an advanced government in a peaceful and successful democratic country, enabling citizens to fulfill their full potential for the betterment of the society as a whole.

For many years, scientists studied the nervous (neuro) and immune systems as if they were separate and unique. But over the last twenty years, research has demonstrated that this is a misunderstanding. The truth is that these two systems are intimately entwined to such an extent that they might be considered as one. Research now demonstrates with increasing complexity how nerve and immune cells work hand in hand. They share many common traits, including memory and plasticity. They speak the same language, share similar functions, and in many places are physically attached.

With that said, I want to give you a brief overview of each system separately, but you'll see how they work together in harmony.

THE IMMUNE SYSTEM

Your immune system's primary function is to help create and manage a peaceful society. It fashions and maintains a safe environment where other cells can thrive and carry out their roles in making your body work.

In addition to this housekeeping role, immune cells undertake functions as diverse as isolating and fighting off infections, through the formation and consolidation of memories in the brain. They influence your metabolism and energy levels, the storage of fat, and the health and function of many types of muscles. Finally, they direct the cells that perform maintenance and repair throughout the body. They also have a key policing role, preserving the peace among different groups of cells with their competing needs and agendas, including the diverse cell types of their own team.

Part of the immune system functions as a modern military force made up of different branches and sub-branches, with skills and capabilities specific to each. A command structure with generals and officers coordinates operations. Many different types of soldiers are trained for specific roles and missions. There are fighting branches assisted by a myriad of support divisions traveling through complex systems of blood and lymphatic vessels. "Scientist" cells pull apart viruses, bacteria, and other organisms, working out how best to kill them. Chemists and engineering cells manufacture toxic chemicals and specialty weapons like antibodies.

The marrow in your bones and the thymus gland are the primary breeding grounds of these cells. They are trained for their missions all over the body in specialist tissues: the thymus gland, the spleen, the numerous lymph nodes situated throughout your body, and most importantly in the tissues of the wall of the gut, the liver, the airways of your lungs, and beneath your skin.

But the military task, fighting infections and cancer, is only one small part of the immune branch's functions. Immune cells are crucial not only to fight disease and invasion from both outside and inside the body, but also in maintaining the health and normal function of the body's tissues and organs, including your brain.

Thus their main role is much more mundane than fighting wars. These cells are the silent key workers of the body keeping all the systems running smoothly.

This understanding is a new and important shift in immunology thinking.

THE NERVOUS (NEURO) SYSTEM

Now let's talk about the other branch of the neuro-immune system: the nervous system. This is the body's World Wide Web, connecting every part of us through a network of fast and slow fibers transmitting millions of messages per minute.

The central nervous system, composed of the brain and spinal cord, is like the central processor of a supercomputer. Although you hear about artificial intelligence, our current capabilities are dwarfed by the brain. In 2014, Japanese scientists, on what was then the fourth-fastest supercomputer in the world, took forty minutes to accomplish what 1 percent of the brain does in one second. Remarkably, the energy required to run the brain would struggle to keep a small ten-watt light bulb dimly lit! Our brain is literally the pinnacle of millions of years of evolution.

Nerves project from the CNS to reach every part of the body, indeed almost every cell. The primary role of nerve tissue is to collect and send information around the body at very high speeds. It runs very much like an old-fashioned telephone network. Millions of individual wires carry information from specialist sensors to the central processing systems in the spinal cord and the brain. (Given that we are around thirty-five trillion cells, that's a lot of wires!)

The traffic is a two-way system with other fibers carrying signals out, causing muscle fibers to contract, glands to secrete hormones, sweat glands to create sweat, and blood vessels to dilate or contract, altering blood flow through the tissues of the body. Many of these fibers are heading to various components of the immune system! These connections include clusters of immune cells, such as in lymph nodes, or those found in the gut wall right down to individual cells in many cases.

As these nerve fibers come together, they form larger and larger units, becoming cables of wires, and finally trunks containing tens of thousands of individual nerve fibers. The longest nerve in the body runs from the tip of your big toe to the base of your spinal cord, which ends at the level of the lower curve in your back—around forty inches in length. The transmission rates can be as fast as 270 mph in fibers supplying muscles, down to one mile per hour in those dealing with some body functions. That means that a nerve impulse or message traveling from the toe to the spine takes around one thousandth of a second.

Individual nerve cells have unique functions. There are whole groups of them that have specialist sensors whose job it is to recognize threats to the well-being of the body. These might be invaders (viruses, bacteria, and fungi) or your own cells that are worn out, sick themselves, or cancer cells. For a long time, we thought this ability was confined to the cells of the immune system. Now we know that some nerves are equally capable of recognizing invaders and threats, setting the immune system to work. These threats include chemicals and molecules that in excess are harmful to the body as a whole. No surprise that sugar, certain proteins, and some fats are included in this category.

An important takeaway from the connected nature of the two systems is that when the nervous system is out of balance, the immune system will follow. The converse is equally true: an unbalanced immune system leads to an unbalanced nervous system. Or think of it this way: your nervous system includes your brain, so an unhappy brain equals an unhappy immune system—and an unhappy immune system leads to an unhappy brain.

The Endocrine System

If the nervous system is the high-speed World Wide Web of the body, the endocrine system is that which sets the background tone or mood. It is made up of a collection of cells and glands, which produce a host of different chemicals that influence the way the body works in a slower fashion.

Most people have heard of thyroxine from the thyroid gland in your neck, or the sex hormones estrogen from the ovaries and testosterone from the testes, and of course cortisol, the so-called stress hormone from your adrenal glands. But these are just the tip of the iceberg. There are over two hundred different hormones and hormone-like peptides that circulate in our body. For example, grehlin from the stomach tells us that we are hungry. Insulin and glucagon control sugar levels in the body, and leptin controls fat.

The role of all these hormones is to set the background operating level of much of the body's machinery, in the same way that a thermostat sets the temperature in a house or a dimmer switch controls the light level and ambiance of the room.

These hormones regulate our basic metabolic rate and levels of arousal and sexual desire, and they influence the way our gut digests food or rests. They can act locally, especially in the gut where they control the secretion of digestive enzymes and the function of the gallbladder, or on far-distant structures like the brain, telling it that we have eaten enough.

Yet again the neuro-immune system appears in the story. Our hormone-producing cells, whether operating as individual cells in the lining layer of the gut wall or as a group of cells in a gland like the thyroid, are under the influence of the nervous system. Furthermore, many immune cells and nerve cells not only carry receptors for hormones but are themselves able to manufacture many of the different hormones typically made by more specialist endocrine cells. The effect is pop-up micro-glands producing hormones confined to very localized and often microscopic spaces.

One crucial hormone is cortisol. This master hormone, which is elevated in stress—when the body or mind perceives itself being under attack—has far-reaching effects on every system in the body, including the neuro-immune system itself. These effects are beneficial in the short term, but too much cortisol produced by chronic stress has profoundly damaging effects across the body.

Melatonin, the sleep hormone, is another important hormone. Long associated with sleep regulation, melatonin is now understood to influence many cells in the immune system—and several make melatonin themselves. This hormone has roles in not only protecting peripheral nerves but also modifying their behavior, for example in pain modulation. Alterations in light exposure, which affects melatonin production, not only lead to disturbed and disrupted sleep but negatively affect the neuro-immune system. This in part explains the link between quality sleep patterns and health.

Before we move on to consider other conditions that come about through the disruption of one or more of these systems, there is one more area of the body that we must visit, and it is perhaps the most crucial to understanding health: the gut.

The Gut

The nerves in the gut make up your second brain. It is every bit as, and indeed arguably *more*, complicated than the brain in our head.

Additionally, around 85 percent of your immune cells are located in the gut wall and liver. The gut also contains around thirty hormones and over one hundred bioactive peptides, which act as chemical messengers, influencing both local and distant tissues by directly acting on nerves and immune cells.

This almost incomprehensibly complex matrix of over one hundred million individual neurons and their supporting cells are part of an amazing system. A structure that not only allows for the passage of food along the intestine in an orderly fashion, but, in conjunction with immune and endocrine cells in the wall of the gut, orchestrate the immensely complicated task of digesting and absorbing that food. All while preventing the entry of toxic substances, bacteria, and other microorganisms.

The gut is also the location of one of our most important "organs," the microbiota or microbial colony, which shares our journey through life. This colony is so important that it is truly the center of our personal universe. If it's not healthy, we are not healthy. Fact! (More on the microbiota in a bit.)

The gut is a twenty-two-foot-long tube starting at the mouth and finishing at your anus. We pour eights liters of fluid into it every day to digest food—the equivalent of one-quarter of all the water in our body! We reabsorb 97 percent of that water in the large intestine. Attached to the gut are the liver, gallbladder, and pancreas.

Critical to health is the border that lies between the contents of the gut and our inner world. This border is like tiles on a floor—a thin, single-layered barrier with grout lines between. The grout lines seal the gaps between the cells, which is crucial to border integrity because in a healthy gut, substances can enter only by traveling through the cells rather than between them. In a disease situation, the grout lines can fail, and this can lead to a "leaky" gut barrier and all sorts of problems, including a leaky blood-brain barrier (more on this later).

· ·

If you laid out your gut on a flat surface, it would cover an area the size of a tennis court.

· ·

The gut lining, the *epithelium,* is coated by a thick layer of mucus. This protective mucus is bi-layered like a sponge cake. In and on the outer layer live our *microbiota,* but the inner layer is impenetrable to them and forms a barrier separating them from the surface cells. Just as the grout lines between cells must remain intact to protect us, so must the mucus coating maintain its healthy, two-layer structure.

If this border is breached, bacteria and lots of other molecules can enter the body, and this has serious consequences.

Maintaining the integrity of this seemingly innocuous barrier is possibly one of the single most important goals for ensuring health and preventing sickness. As you read on, I will show you how.

In just a moment, we are going to take a closer look at the helpful friends living in the gut, but first, we have to clear something up about germs.

"GERMS"

If you are like most people, you have been raised to believe that bacteria, fungi, and viruses are all "dirty" and dangerous. Some of these so-called germs can indeed cause pneumonia, sinus infections, strep throat, meningitis, urinary infections, and skin infections including boils (bacteria), head colds, most sore throats, flu, pneumonia, bronchitis, and many childhood illnesses with rashes (viruses), such as ringworm, athlete's foot, and jock itch (fungi). But these diseases are caused by a minuscule part of the microbial world.

The story further goes that to be healthy and well you need to live in a germ-free environment. In fact, the truth is totally the opposite. In our natural state, we have evolved surrounded by all sorts of microorganisms. Most of these so-called germs are actually beneficial to us; without them we would be unhealthy and unable to survive. We need to be constantly exposed to a wide variety of organisms to keep our immune systems robust and healthy.

· ·

A walk in nature, especially a woodland, boosts your immune system for several days. Camp out overnight in the same setting and this becomes weeks.

· ·

This does not mean that it is appropriate to live in a filthy environment without sanitation and clean running water, but nor should we attempt to sterilize our surroundings. In fact, we should strive for the opposite. Children need to get dirty and play in the mud. Other than our kitchens, cooking surfaces, and bathrooms, our homes should be clean but not sterile. Gardening, a walk in the woods, stroking pets and other animals are all activities that are good for us. Part of the benefit is due to contact with microorganisms.

Far from being dangerous, the invisible microbial world assists us in so many ways. Besides protecting us from disease, soil organisms—mainly bacteria and fungi—allow our food plants to grow with high levels of nutrients that benefit us.

So why am I mentioning this here? Because these microorganisms did not just evolve around us. They evolved with us and indeed inside us. Arguably, *we* evolved around them. Bacteria and fungi made up the first living organisms in evolutionary history. They have been around 3.5 billion years compared to 300,000 for modern man, which is many millions of years longer than us.

The microbiota, also called the microbiome, is the name given to the various organisms that share our body. Although you may find this difficult to accept, there are more bacteria cells than human cells inside you!

Every part of our body—and I mean *every* part—has its own colony of microorganisms. The master colony lives in your intestine, your gut, and is by far the largest, with probably sixty-five to one hundred trillion bacteria, weighing about three pounds—the same weight as a human brain. This colony has the greatest number of species and the greatest diversity. It is one of the densest bacterial ecosystems on the planet. The colony produces a myriad of chemicals that influence how our entire body operates. Its health is critical to our health and, in the same way as we need to protect nature and our environment for human societies to flourish, we need to strive for good health to provide an appropriate habitat for our microbiota to thrive.

. . . .

The importance of the microbiota in your overall health cannot be overstated. It is increasingly clear that it is possibly the most important "organ" in your body, which influences every system that runs us.

. . . .

You inherit your microbiota colony from your mother, the rest of the family, and pets (especially dogs) living in the house. The colonization of the gut occurs during the first three years of life. (This is one of the reasons why antibiotics given to young children are so damaging to long-term health.) The mode of your birth, whether vaginal delivery or C-section, gives rise to very different colonies and, ultimately, life outcomes.

Once you have inherited the basic colony, the structure is predicated by your lifestyle; it's primarily your diet, but it also includes your amount of exercise, sleep, and levels of stress. Your environment, city or country, and the number of pets and animals you come in contact with also have a profound influence. (On the whole, the closer you get to nature, the better off you are.)

Finally, you can think of the nerves and immune cells in the gut wall as the means by which the microbiota communicates with the rest of us, in particular our brain.

THE ROLE OF THE MICROBIOTA

The microbiota has a significant and important role in managing not only your immune system's initial development, health, and overall function during your whole life, but it also influences the development of the central nervous system (brain) during childhood and its day-to-day function during your lifespan. In addition, it regulates and controls many key metabolic processes in the body. As you can see, the microbiota influences every aspect of the running of the human meta-organism.

> This includes the food you crave. Changing the gut colony composition changes your food cravings! It takes about three months for this to happen.

One of our primary defenses against infection is found in the microbial colonies around the body. In some cases, disease-causing bacteria and fungi are already present as part of the resident community in the very same location in which they cause disease. However, they are kept in their place by competition with other inhabiting bacteria and fungi.

Infections occur due to a breakdown of the local ecology and a dysbiosis of the resident microbiota, which allows the overgrowth of one particular strain that, if present in sufficient number, can cause disease. For example, many of us have the strep bacteria in the back of our throat that causes strep throat, but very few of us get this condition. The resident colony of 200 other species and our immune system keeps the numbers of strep bacteria in check.

So you have to think of infections in a new way. Many represent an imbalance but not a novel invasion. Being healthy and fit helps maintain the balance and protects you from infection.

The local microbiota also appears to influence the local immune system's response to any imbalance. It not only alerts our immune cells that there is an overgrowth of a potentially aggressive species, but it also assists in directing the correct reaction based on the type of organism. It also appears that it can actively take part in the defense process by producing an array of antimicrobial molecules active against "invaders."

This is one of the reasons why antibiotics need to be used with extreme caution. They have the potential to damage these normal protective mechanisms by throwing the system into even deeper disarray, both in the short and long term. Antibiotics, of course, can be critical when the infection is out of control, but they have the capacity to significantly damage the microbiota's ability to defend itself and the human body. The use of antibiotics comes with a price!

This influence of the resident microbiota upon "infections" is not just confined to controlling bacteria and fungi overgrowth. It also includes viruses. It has been shown that your response to the flu virus is in part influenced by the quality of your gut microbiota. We know that several bacteria produce antiviral molecules that are active against the COVID-19 virus.

To be healthy, you require diverse, balanced, and healthy bacterial colonies in every part of your body, but especially in your gut. As part of the aging process, we seem to lose the richness of species in the gut with profound consequences. Keeping bacterial species diversity as you age, with a broad and varied diet, is key to slowing this process. Unfortunately, as we get older, the opposite tends to happen. We become narrower in food choices and cooking skills. This is a significant issue in institutions, such as care homes.

Specific colonies of organisms are influenced by their environment. If you change the environment, you change the community structure. Every aspect of how you choose to live your life influences your microbial colonies' health: the type of shampoo, soap, or perfume you use; whether your house is "sterile" or just clean; how much stress, both physical and emotional, you are exposed to. Of course, it also includes whether you exercise, are primarily sedentary, and if you get a good amount of quality sleep. Nonetheless, nothing influences the colonies more than the food available to them locally. Modern lifestyles and environments have played havoc with the ecological balance of this system.

The bacterial colonies also alter your response to many medications, including modern cancer therapies. They influence immune responses in autoimmune disease, including eczema and asthma. Increasingly, we recognize that they modify the functions of your nervous system, including the brain.

The intestinal colony has an enormous impact not only over our digestive processes and general metabolism but also our mental health. It influences our mood and plays a role in motivation and psychological well-being, as well as disease. We have demonstrated that we can transfer anxiety between mice with fecal transplants. There is strong evidence that probiotics and diet can influence both mood and emotional reactions in humans. Finally, in this realm of gut-brain connectivity, we are beginning to understand the mechanisms behind the roles that the microbiota plays in a diverse group of psychologically challenging syndromes, including autism spectrum disorders and Functional Pain syndromes.

In short, the bacterial colony in your gut (and to a lesser extent other sites) influences every aspect of your life.

There are two basic extremes in gut microbiota: One is a colony that causes inflammation not only locally in the gut wall but also systemically, throughout the whole body. The other end of the spectrum is a microbiota that is anti-inflammatory in nature. This, of course, is the one you want.

"What is inflammation, and why do I want an anti-inflammatory microbiota?" you ask? Let's take a closer look.

Inflammation

Inflammation is a process that can be both beneficial and destructive.

Inflammation is a single name for a complex series of neuro-immune and neuro-endocrine events that, combined, allows the body to protect itself from damage, warding off attacks by invaders or rogue cancer cells, or healing tissues damaged by injury.

Sometimes this is a double-edged sword. What works to the body's benefit in saving us from infections, cancer, or trauma can become a significant destructive force if it continues long term.

Acute inflammation is how we protect ourselves from infection and injury. *Chronic* inflammation, however, is the root of all noninfectious diseases. It is the process that causes arthritis, heart disease, high blood pressure, diabetes, depression, and dementia. Chronic inflammation is the leading cause of decreased healthspan (or the amount of your life lived in good health) and life expectancy.

Chronic inflammation is influenced by many things: your lifestyle, your life experiences including those of your childhood, your attitudes, beliefs, and the health of your microbiota.

. . . .

The take-home message from this entire book is that you have direct control over your lifestyle and your thoughts; indeed, these are the only things that you have control over. By deciding how you want to live and experience life with all its challenges profoundly influences your internal world. Thus, to a great extent, you decide your destiny.

. . . .

We need to control the level of this chronic or background inflammation because it is this slow, often unnoticed, process that ages us prematurely and destroys our physical and mental health.

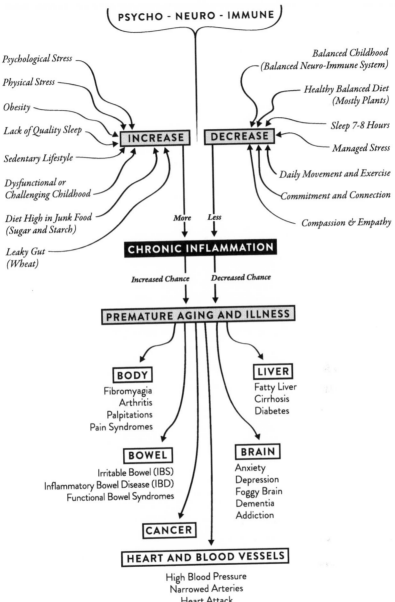

There are three simple blood markers of inflammation that your doctor can easily measure, and you should ask for one of them to be checked as part of any annual labs. C-reactive protein (CRP) is the easiest and perhaps the most used marker of both acute and chronic background inflammation. It is a protein made in the liver and fat cells, produced when we have an infection or there is damage to the body. Levels rise quickly with acute threats but will fall equally fast after you get better. In the absence of acute infection or tissue damage, elevated levels of CRP are a pretty good marker of chronic inflammation. You should monitor and follow your CRP levels. I suggest patients ask for high-sensitive CRP (hs-CRP) as it is more accurate at low levels. Erythrocyte Sedimentation Rate (ESR) and plasma viscosity are also good tests of inflammation.

It makes sense that if we recognize that chronic inflammation is the cause of almost all noninfectious disease, then we should aim to have the lowest level of CRP. Doctors tend to use this test in the setting of acute infections or acute inflammatory disease. However, if you are tracking your "Wellness Score," (as you'll see in Chapter 9) then although it has limitations, it can be a useful marker.

Away from the brain, metabolic stress in the form of high cholesterol (hyperlipidemia) or high sugar levels (hyperglycemia), as occurs in diabetes or after a very sugary meal, leads to increased neuro-immune, system-driven "background" inflammation, and the end result of this process is slow and continuing damage to the tissues of the body. Here we link the process by which poor diets with abnormal loads of nutrients directly affect your immune system in a harmful manner. (We will discuss how to reverse some of this harm in Chapter 3.)

Food-driven dysfunction also causes the formation of inflamed, thickened plaques in the lining of blood vessels, which causes them to narrow and sometimes block, a disease called atheroma. This, in turn, causes heart attacks, strokes, and erectile dysfunction. This direct effect of nutrients on the immune system explains why levels of inflammation are important in regard to blood vessel health and heart disease, not cholesterol levels alone. Further, it explains how even short episodes of excess and unhealthy eating habits can precipitate catastrophic events, such as heart attacks or strokes.

Additionally, we know that having too much belly fat, also called intra-abdominal fat, increases inflammation in the body and losing weight decreases it. As you now understand, this chronic low-level inflammation leads to accelerated aging of the body and mind, as well as chronic disease.

THE GUT AND INFLAMMATION

Think of the intestine wall like a border between two countries, with the neuro-immune system on one side and the microbial colony on the other. We need trade and products to go both ways across the border, but it is all very carefully managed by both sides.

The way in which this border control system in your gut wall operates has enormous implications on your general health. It plays a significant role in dictating the amount of background inflammation throughout the body. What happens in your intestine wall influences every other part of your body, including your brain. This is in part because many cell types of the immune system are able to migrate all over the body, partly because of chemical messaging from those that remain, and partly due to a direct-link superhighway between the gut and the brain called the vagus nerve.

Bottom line: what happens in the gut does not stay in the gut.

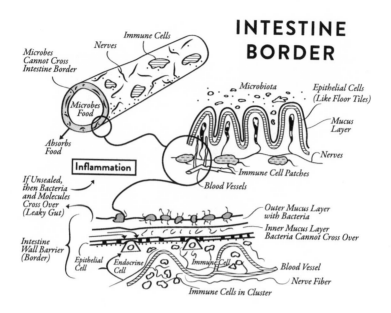

So why does this matter? The answer is that if the barrier between the bacterial colony in the gut and the neuro-immune system lining the gut wall malfunctions, we create an inflammatory reaction that spreads. It is now clear that to a great extent our body's background level of chronic inflammation is set in the gut wall. It appears that many if not most inflammatory and autoimmune diseases start here, and in those that don't, this system becomes involved.

It has been proposed that one key ingredient in our contemporary diet that causes this breakdown in the barrier is related to the consumption of large amounts of modern wheat. This is the story of gluten. All of us are, to some degree, wheat intolerant. When gluten is digested in our gut, we produce polypeptide chains that up-regulate a protein called zonulin. This protein opens gates in the grout lines between the cells that line the gut—gates that are normally closed. When the gates open, molecules and bacterial products and indeed occasionally bacteria themselves that are supposed to remain in the gut lumen meet the immune system in the gut wall. The effect is inflammation and sensitization, which has the potential to lead to autoimmune diseases like rheumatoid arthritis, diabetes, MS, and others. This is why there is an argument that suggests that anybody who has a chronic illness or an autoimmune disease should consider significantly reducing or actually removing wheat and wheat-based products from their diet, at least on a temporary basis.

Further, we are now beginning to recognize that the breakdown of the gut barrier is sometimes associated with a failure of the so-called blood-brain barrier. This allows molecules and immune cells that normally cannot access the brain directly to enter with significant consequences to the functioning of the central nervous system. This produces the experience known to many people with gut health issues as the foggy brain.

Pain

Like inflammation, pain can be both a blessing and—for many—a curse.

Pain evolved to keep us safe, warn us that something is wrong, teach us how to interact with the environment, and let us know when we need to withdraw and rest. Most of the time, that is exactly how it works.

However, just as the immune system cells and the neuro-immune system can go wrong, so can the pain management and pain perception system. This leads to all sorts of unpleasant and complex pain syndromes.

Pain perception is not simply a matter of the wiring of the circuits of nerve fibers and the behavior of immune cells. Two other key components that influence pain are memory and emotion. Your psychological makeup, dictated in part by your developmental experience during childhood, has a profound effect on how you experience pain.

Sometimes the system develops in an abnormal way because of this modeling by its environment. Thus it might come as no surprise that people who had difficult childhoods, whether from trauma, sickness, neglect, or abuse, are much more prone to developing abnormal pain responses. This is due to the same processes that make them more likely to suffer from chronic anxiety and depression along with chronic illness.

Most of us know someone with fibromyalgia, and between 10 percent and 20 percent of us will experience irritable bowel syndrome (IBS) at some period in our life. These painful conditions are extremely debilitating and horribly frustrating because doctors have no tools to measure where the system has gone wrong or where the fault lies in the very complex neuro-immune system.

One thing is for sure: although we perceive pain in our head, because pain is a construct of the brain, this does not mean that it is "all in your head." These syndromes are complex neuro-immune illnesses, and they are very real from an anatomical and physiological point of view. We just have not figured out the details or how to locate the defect.

However, even though we lack precision in our diagnostic tools to locate the exact fault, or more likely faults, we can mold the system through various behaviors. How to do this? Read on.

The Mind-Body Connection

The artificial barriers of the last century of western thinking, where people treated the mind and body as being separate, are falling. Many of the commonly recognized connections between our emotional and physical health are being explained on a biological basis teased out by science.

The relatively new discipline of *psychoneuroimmunology* is beginning to demonstrate the profound effects that your mental (psychological) well-being has on your physical health by altering your nervous and immune systems. The closely related discipline of *psychoneuroendocrinology*, the study of how stress affects the many hormones in our body, has been around longer and is much more widely accepted.

When was the last time you went to a medical practitioner for a checkup? Even if you don't go, most people understand that it is a good idea. But have you ever considered going to see a clinical psychologist for a mental health check? My guess is never. Yet you probably should. Paying attention to your psychological and emotional well-being could literally save your life.

Most people think that psychology is the study of personality and mood, but this is incorrect. One of the key roles of the nervous system, along with the immune system, is to measure and sense what is going on around us and indeed inside us, building an ever-changing model of our internal and external world. This model is then used to produce reactions and actions, which include not only movement and behaviors like eating, but also emotions, moods, and memories. The study of how this all happens is called psychology.

So when people talk about going to see a psychologist about mental health problems, they are talking about a fairly small part of psychology—the field of clinical psychology, which deals with thoughts, behaviors, and moods. As you can see, psychology is much more than that. The important thing to understand is that all of this is run by and originates from the neuro-immune system.

PSYCHONEUROIMMUNOLOGY

The world of psychoneuroimmunology and psychoneuroendocrinology is where scientific enquiry demonstrates the importance of mental well-being on our health. These closely related research disciplines explore the influence of emotional states (like depression or happiness) and nervous system activities (like stress) on immune system functions; how these psychological states relate to the onset and progression of disease and aging.

Researchers now have techniques and technologies to measure the biological processes that demonstrate how the mind and body meet, how they influence each other, and indeed how functionally they have to be considered to be one entity, not two.

Have you ever wondered why, when you get the flu or have a physical injury, you often become anxious, "blue," or even depressed? You are not imagining things. It is in part an adaptive response, and in part an immune, cell-mediated inflammatory process arising from the reaction to the infection or injury. Just as what happens in the gut does not stay in the gut, what happens at infection or injury sites spreads around the body. It is a process common to many illnesses, although there is some individual variation in the degree to which people experience it.

When an animal becomes unwell, it shows some very typical behaviors you will recognize if you have a cat or dog: they stop eating, go find a quiet spot, withdraw from the world, and lay still. This is sickness behavior. If you are human and behave like this, we label you as being depressed. However, when you are unwell, this sickness behavior is *normal*. Withdrawing from the world is part of how we heal. For our ancestors who lived in a harsh environment, full of danger with the constant risk of injury and infection, sickness behavior probably increased chances of survival. Being still, quiet, and fasting improved the chance of healing and mending. It also perhaps reflects the neuro-immune system's attempt to calm the sympathetic nervous system, which we now recognize—if in overdrive—inhibits immune cell activity. Noradrenalin (the sympathetic system's neurotransmitter) might save your life in the short term, with fight or flight, but you can have too much of a good thing. It, along with the hormone cortisol, suppresses immune cell mobility and killing capabilities. This is not helpful if you are relying on this system to heal you and keep you alive.

This adaptive behavior and depressed feelings typically occur anytime you are in a threatening and stressful situation. This reaction is strongest in defeat stress, the type we get when we are facing something that truly endangers us, either physically or mentally. Relatively short-term stress associated with a challenge, say to perform better by studying for a test, produces a subtly different stress response, which in fact is beneficial.

Sickness behavior is related to high levels of both acute and chronic inflammation. Inflammation anywhere in the body leads to neuro-immune cells sending chemical and nerve signals to the brain. Thus, illness or injury has a profound effect on your brain. This is a two-way street: mental stress and illness changes the immune system and makes you much more prone to all sorts of physical illnesses, including high blood pressure, diabetes, obesity, autoimmune diseases, and cancer. Conversely, physical illness makes you much more prone to mental ill-health, including anxiety.

This explains why mental well-being, or its opposite, distress, which are primary functions of your nervous system, has such profound effects on your immune system's function. Equally, we now understand that chemicals and messaging molecules produced by immune cells directly influence the behavior of nerve cells, including those that are involved in learning, memory, and mood.

Psychological stress leads to chronic inflammation and maladapted responses to infection and tumor cells. It's why stress kills you. Equally, infections, trauma, and cancer all lead to neurological changes, often in the form of altered sleep patterns, depression, and anxiety.

What is important to understand here is that depression, anxiety, and indeed pain are not always diseases. They are the neuro-immune system's expression of being out of balance. The route to mending them is not just giving a medication alone (which might influence a few chemical pathways, often does not work, and indeed can do harm, such as increased risk of suicide) but to take an approach that influences the thousands of chemical pathways operating at any one moment in time. This requires treating the whole person primarily by changing behavior.

From a practical point of view, the significance of this is that we need to move away from a system-based approach to health and consider the wider interactions of all cells in the body, including the microbiota. Health and illness are multifactorial and controlled by our microorganism colonies and the neuro-immune system, which are in turn molded by our physical and social environment and lifestyle. Maladaptation in any part of the system leads to a loss of balance in the whole system and to disease. To provide meaningful sickness care requires that we truly address health, which is the state of complete physical, mental, and social well-being.

Your To-Do List

- Have an annual checkup and ask your healthcare provider to measure your HbA1c (average sugar level) and vitamin D levels along with your standard tests.

- At your annual checkup, have your healthcare provider assess chronic inflammation by measuring your C-Reactive Protein (CRP). (I request patients ask for high-sensitive CRP (hs-CRP) as it is more accurate at low levels.)

- Consider also scheduling a checkup with a psychologist. You don't have to be unwell to see a psychologist. However, if you are physically ill, then I would suggest this should be a vital component of your treatment plan due to the intimate link between your brain and body. Your personality, attitudes, and approach to life matters and influences your physical health more than you realize.

- Read Part II of this book to learn more about diet, exercise, sleep, Me-Time, and stress reduction for whole-body health.

- Fill in your Wellness Score sheet (see Chapter 9) on a regular basis.

The gut, with its resident neuro-immune system and microbiota, is the center of the human universe and needs to be carefully tended like a garden. Additionally, as we have learned, stress will age and kill you prematurely if you don't take action to manage it. Both stress and your gut influence the amount of inflammation in your body.

Now that you have this foundational learning in place, Part II will show you how to maintain both your body and your mind for improved health and better living.

PART II

THE FIVE
ELEMENTS

· · · · · · · · · · · · · · · · · · · ·

CHAPTER 3

DECODING DIET

· ·

The last few months of my mother's life were challenging. She and my sister lived together on a small hill farm in the west of England. Typically, they ate a straightforward and healthy diet. In the UK, we call it meat and two veg, with potatoes on the side. (And the portion of meat is small!)

When my mother became ill at the very end of her life, one of the things that went by the wayside was the preparation of real food. They started to eat premade meals from the supermarket, though they were of good quality. My sister thought they were doing okay on this diet, until she switched back to her regular home-cooked meals as things settled. Within a few days, she noticed a significant difference in how she felt.

It was a clear lesson: home-prepared, natural, fresh food is best.

A Discussion about Diet

The whole discussion about diet leaves me completely perplexed. We spend millions of dollars figuring out why we have an obesity and diabetes pandemic along with numerable other noninfectious diseases when the answer is right in front of our eyes. The truth is that we eat too much and too often. We consume too many carbs and an excess of sugar, and we don't eat enough fiber. In short, most of us live on highly processed, manufactured "food," best described as junk. Many add insult to injury by consuming sugary drinks and too much alcohol.

How did we get here? It's all about the food industry, a drug called sugar, a substance called salt, and of course politics and economics, along with clever marketing. As the saying goes, "follow the money."

It's not your fault that you overeat. The real issue is the clever marketing of cheap, scientifically manufactured foods aimed at satisfying natural "addictions."

The average daily calorie intake in the US has increased by 25 percent since 1950, although interestingly in the UK, another country plagued by obesity and overweight issues, it declined slightly in the last few years while weights continue to spiral upwards (read on to discover why). The quantities of protein and fat consumed have remained relatively constant, so the increase is almost exclusively due to the addition of calorie-rich sweeteners. In other words, sugars.

From an evolutionary standpoint, it is easy to understand why the brain might crave foods containing sugar. In the world of our ancestors, where obtaining sufficient nutrients and energy was their primary challenge, sugar from honey provided an excellent source of energy to build fat stores, and our brain developed circuits that would drive us to seek it out.

And we can't forget about salt. The human body is primarily a bag full of saline—a solution of salt and water. To ensure that the body's chemistry functions correctly, we need salt to maintain an exact level of salinity or salt-water balance. Because we cannot make salt, it is a critical part of our diet.

Not surprisingly, our body has a powerful hardwired natural craving for both salt and sugar. The food manufacturing industry has recognized this and exploited it to improve sales of their products—at our expense. It's sugar and salt that make junk food so yummy and addictive. Around 75 percent of all US barcoded food products contain added sugars, and increasingly many, especially beverages, contain both added sugar and salt. This includes so-called fresh meats.

Equally important is not only what is put in your food, but what is left out. An essential ingredient in a healthy diet is fiber. Relevant to the food industry is that increased fiber in food means a shorter shelf life, more energy to cook, and more effort to eat. So if you want people to buy and consume your product, remove the fiber. The trouble is that this is a big problem for your health.

As humans, we are flexitarian omnivores, which means that we are adaptable in our dietary requirements. Humans have managed to colonize almost every land-based habitat on the planet. We have survived in places as diverse as tropical rain forests, dry savannah plains, and the frozen north. The only reason we have been able to do so is that we are adaptable in our dietary, and to a lesser extent nutritional, needs. We are omnivorous in that we are able to eat anything and *flexivorous* in that we can eat whatever is around us right now to sustain us.

But this does not include the multitude of chemical additives and ingredient mixes in modern manufactured foods.

What happens internally when we eat these junk foods? As you learned in Chapter 2, the body ages due to chronic inflammatory damage, and chronic inflammation is to a great extent driven by your diet.

Food is potentially inflammatory. The western diet is very inflammatory. This is a direct and measurable effect due to its influence on the microbiota and neuro-immune system, which evolved to be "fed" natural foods in their original state.

This inflammation arises from the immune cells in the gut wall. Diet influences the intestinal bacterial colony, which in turn affects your gut wall's border integrity and underlying neuro-immune system. Thus, what you eat plays a significant part in dictating the amount of chronic inflammation in your body. As you have learned, what happens in the gut does not stay in the gut. As you will see later, some foods promote inflammation while others actively suppress it.

Arguably, your diet is perhaps the most critical element of being well. If you wish to retain or regain your health, you almost certainly need to change your eating habits. Cutting back and ultimately removing certain foods is the key to success.

It's quite straightforward: stop eating junk and snack foods. Yup, I'm not going to apologize. It's a hard truth, but most people are sick, don't feel well, and are overweight. It's because they overeat and mostly junk.

One thing I know for sure: in all the years that I have been advising patients and helping them improve their health, I have never—and I mean *never*—had a person tell me they felt worse when they removed junk food from their menu and replaced it with natural, properly prepared foods. The universal feedback from 100 percent of them is that they just feel better.

. . . .

If you gain nothing else from this book, I hope you will give up all processed and junk foods, including breads, pastries, cakes, and cookies for thirty to sixty days. Find out what it feels like to eat the way that we and our gut bacterial colony evolved to eat.

. . . .

This is a long chapter, but that is intentional because of just how vitally important your diet is to your health. First, we'll look at some of the things we eat—fat, sugar, fiber—and how they affect our bodies. Then we'll discuss what, how, and even *when* you should eat for better health.

When people ask me what to eat, my response is to borrow and paraphrase Michael Pollan's brilliant line, "Eat real food, mostly plants, and not too much." In fact, we can use that statement to break up the parts of this chapter.

Let's dive in.

Eat Real Food

The only healthy diet is one made up of real food.

Very early in our evolutionary history, we learned to process food. We have chopped it, ground it, dried it, fermented, pickled it, and ultimately cooked it. But it was always recognizable when the process of modifying it was started. It kept its original, basic form. We may have mixed different food sources on a plate, but we did not blend them into each other at a basic level.

The food manufacturing industry, on the other hand, takes real, whole food, dries it, grinds it up into a powder, and mixes it all together in countless ways to make new food. They add chemical ingredients to change taste, texture, and color, and all with a single goal: make it more enticing and easier to consume. The end result? To increase their profits. This is not real food.

Real food is located on the outside wall of the supermarket, in the produce, meat, and dairy sections. You find it in farm stores and farmers' markets. You also find it in your own garden. It is recognizable. It looks like an egg, or a piece of meat, or a plant. It does not come in a can or a box, and it does not have a list of ingredients, or indeed health warnings, attached to it.

Importantly, real food comes as a complete and balanced package. Real food is made by nature. It contains many different components and chemicals, but unlike manufactured foods, the constituents are in balance. Most plant-based foods contain tens and often hundreds of different molecules and chemicals. We and our gut bacteria evolved with these natural blends, and it's how we are supposed to eat.

Patients constantly ask me about different named diets. So let me address a few of the common ones.

Historically, the *Atkins diet* promoted low refined carbohydrates and high protein and fat intake, inducing ketosis and weight loss. After an induction phase of several weeks, carbs are reintroduced in the form of fruits and vegetables. Over the years, this concept has evolved into the paleo-type diet, and indeed, studies support its effectiveness.

At the other extreme, *Dr. Ornish* proposed a very low-fat, lacto-ovo-vegetarian diet. I, along with many others, do not believe that low-fat intake is healthy in the long term. In spite of the current and ongoing fixation with cholesterol, fat is a critical component in a human diet.

High fat, moderate to low protein, low carb: this has been labeled the *keto diet* since the 1920s and comes from a history of therapeutic use in children with brain cancer. Again, there are different schools of thought in the details, but the main thing is that one is exclusively using fat as a fuel source and not glucose at all. So the carbohydrate intake is low enough that ketones are produced in the liver. This keeps the person in a fat-burning state, whether that's from what they consume or their own stores. It promotes metabolic flexibility and keeps your fat stores in check.

The concept of *intermittent fasting* is one of the newer ones on the block. Removing all food intake for more than sixteen to eighteen hours forces the body to start using its fat stores, pushing most individuals into ketosis. It's entirely normal for humans to miss meals, so, to my mind, this is not really a diet; it's how we should eat. There are multiple variations. For example, many people have found it easiest to adhere to a sixteen-hour "overnight" fast by missing breakfast, and an eight-hour eating window during the day. Others prefer the 4–2 formula, four days free eating, two days full fast. It's tough, but it works and is probably how our forefathers ate much of the time.

The *paleo diet* is a mash-up of ideas, including some from Atkins. It encourages us to eat in the same way as our distant ancestors. The only issue for me is that it seems fictitious. The foods available were so different from today that it's perhaps a "romantic" version of reality. But having made this dismissive statement, I am 100 percent supportive of the idea of eating whole foods prepared and cooked from their original state. So it gets a thumbs-up in several categories.

Vegans do not eat any foods that come from animals or fish. Vegan diets are best supplemented with B12 and other nutrients that are scarce in exclusively plant-based foods. There is also evidence that vegans have a higher risk of hemorrhagic stroke than others, further supporting the idea that it may risk dietary deficiencies in particular nutrients.

Before every vegan throws this book in the trash, let me say that I am not proposing that you cannot survive and be extremely healthy on a vegan diet. But to be successful, you must know what you're doing and typically be prepared to use some supplements.

I understand that there are many reasons other than health that would make someone choose to follow this lifestyle. There are environmental and ethical issues that come into play, and I am very sympathetic with these. What I am suggesting is that a *pure* vegan diet is perhaps not the best for most people. If consumed in modest amounts, both dairy products and eggs can be produced ethically and fill the nutrient gap that many vegans and some vegetarians fall into.

What do all these diets have in common? They are based on real food.

The take-home message is that there is no specific human diet. There are many types of foods that one can eat to reach the same endpoint, as the body is truly flexible. However, a highly processed, high-sugar, high-refined carb, high-fat, and low-fiber diet is not a good diet for anyone.

Mostly Plants

When we look at the bacterial colony that lives in our gut, we recognize very different types of bacteria depending upon what we eat.

In simple terms, if you eat a lot of plant food containing a preponderance of fiber, you will have an anti-inflammatory colony, which is helpful and beneficial for your overall health. Diets full of refined carbs, sugars, and large quantities of animal products tend to produce an inflammatory colony—unhelpful for your health.

Variety is beneficial, so it would be best if you chose the widest selection of plant foods available to you. The idea of the *rainbow diet* best encapsulates this. Choose a diet that not only has lots of natural plant-based products in it, but one in which you incorporate as many different colors and types of plants as possible.

Similarly, grains in your diet should be from various sources: rice, traditional grains like oats, spelt, amaranth, quinoa, and very modest amounts of wheat and corn. The latter two, along with soy, have become staples as they are easy to grow, but we are not designed to eat large quantities. Their mass production and consumption have created a myriad of problems for us, the entire food production chain, and our ecosystems.

The idea that modern man needs to eat large amounts of meat and other animal products to remain healthy is unsupported by scientific data. There is a lot of epidemiological information to support the idea that lowering the proportion of animal products from the currently high levels consumed in several western-style diets confers broad health benefits. Some research supports the idea that in many groups, diets high in animal products can promote insulin resistance, diabetes, and metabolic disorders more traditionally associated with high-carb diets. So, although we are omnivores, we are omnivores with a caveat: animal products probably need to be consumed in moderation in most societies.

That said, animal source foods do have very high general nutrition value, and so having *some* animal products on your plate is beneficial. Too much, however, is not good for most of us.

If consumed, animal products should be balanced. For most of us, dairy—meaning milk, cheese, and yogurt—should be kept to moderate amounts. The same goes for meats. There is conflicting evidence supporting the idea that white meat is a great deal better than red meat, but it's a complex issue. One of the best animal protein sources are small, oily fish. Sardines and herring are the two that I recommend and are currently sourced in a sustainable fashion. The other is free-range eggs.

Mix it up. Variety is the spice of life.

And Not a Lot

The reality is that, in our modern culture, equally important to *what* we eat is *how much* we eat. It's too much—and yes, it is that simple.

And there's a reason why: food is available everywhere, in every store, gas/mini-mart station, and clothes shop. If there is a cash register, there is junk food. We have vending machines everywhere.

The result? Look around! We are getting fatter and fatter. The explanation? It really is about calories and, most important, where they come from.

CALORIES AND WEIGHT

The reality is that we consume way too much energy-rich food and, as a result, are way too fat.

What's the solution for many to feel better and be healthier? Lose the excess fat. How to lose fat and reach your genetically programmed weight and body shape? For many of us (but not everyone), the answer is eating the right food and lowering calories. It really is that straight-forward. For most of us who are primarily sedentary, 1,400–1,800 calories per day are sufficient if it is a balanced diet.

All of us have a genetically programmed weight and shape, so note I have written that you should lose excess fat. This is different for everyone. You can be "large" and even carry significant fat on your body and remain healthy and well if it is your genetic makeup.

Between 2010 and 2016, the average weight of American men increased by nearly ten pounds from 189 to 198 pounds, and for women seven pounds from 164 to 171 pounds. Since 1960, the difference is an average gain of around thirty pounds. That's approaching a 20 percent increase in weight! Recall the 25 percent calorie increase I previously mentioned.

This translates into a significant increase in average body mass index (BMI), a measure of the ratio of your height to weight. The goal for most of us should be a BMI between eighteen and twenty-five. Above twenty-five, unless you are an athlete or bodybuilder, you are likely to be overweight. However, BMI does not account for muscle or body type, so although helpful as a rough practical guide, it is not ideal.

AVERAGE BMI VALUES AND WEIGHT OF 18-YEAR-OLD AMERICAN MEN

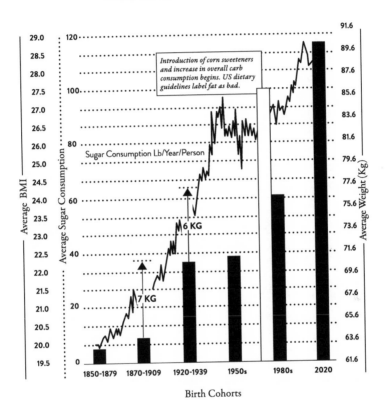

The more important measurement is abdominal circumference, the distance around your tummy one inch above your belly button, which gives some idea of abdominal or visceral fat. This is the critical measurement of your body health.

Average abdominal circumference has also increased since 2000 by more than one inch in men from thirty-nine inches to 40.2 inches in 2016, and two inches in women from 36.3 inches to 38.6 inches. These numbers mean that even in 2000, the average American had an abdominal circumference more than the recommended, and by 2016, it was above that which causes serious health risks.

Regardless of your height or BMI, you should try to lose weight if your tummy size is 37 inches (94 cm) or more for men, and 31.5 inches (80 cm) or more for women. Both of these values seem ridiculously low in 2022, but that's what thirty fewer pounds looks like!

You're at very high risk of some serious health conditions if your tummy size is 40 inches (102 cm) or more for men and 34.5 inches (88 cm) or more for women. Shocked! I bet you are. When I researched this, so was I. But the data supports it.

Before we discuss how to lose that weight, let's look at where those extra calories (and, therefore, extra inches and pounds!) are coming from.

A CALORIE IS NOT A CALORIE

Contrary to the food industry's false claims that all calories are equal, I can firmly and factually state that all calories are not equivalent from a biological point of view.

A calorie is indeed a calorie in thermodynamic science because it is a carefully defined number. Scientists decide how to allocate calories to a certain quantity of a specific food based upon the energy released when that food is burnt in a particular container. But this process has absolutely nothing to do with what goes on in the body. So looking at calories on the side of the packet is at best a guide, and it's often utterly wrong in terms of the way your body works.

Different foods are handled very differently by the body. One calorie from sugar in a soft drink is not the same as one calorie from a carrot. Not even close!

It's much better to think of foods in terms of energy density. This is a physiological concept that, in simple terms, accepts that sugars, starches, and fats have high densities and contain a lot of energy. At the other extreme, fiber derived from plants has a very low energy density. You can eat lots of low-energy-dense food, but you need to be careful of high-density foods.

At the time of writing, the number of calories consumed in the US per day has gone up by an average of 187 calories in men, 335 in women, and 225 in teen boys compared to 1995 levels.

When we look at the breakdown, milk consumption is way down because saturated fat has been labeled as bad. (Although, as it happens, modest amounts of milk fat are more than acceptable to many depending upon your ethnicity, and recent evidence suggests it may even be good for you). Meat and cheese consumption shows minimal or no change. In terms of total fat consumption, it's the same amount in regards to total calorie intake, but the percentage of calories derived from fat in the diet has gone down.

So if calories have gone up, and it has nothing to do with fat, meat, or dairy consumption, where do the extra calories come from? The answer: a significant increase in grains (starches), fruit juice, soft and sports drinks. In short, sugar.

So let's look at sugar in more detail.

SUGAR

Why would the food industry add sugar if we don't need it? The answer, as mentioned previously, is that we are all naturally preprogrammed carb junkies.

If you don't believe me, try giving up carbs. Try completely removing 100 percent of sugar and starches like rice, bread, and potato from your diet! Tough to do, right? It's actually impossible unless you decide to eat a diet of 100 percent fat and pure protein.

The whole carb thing seems to confuse everyone, but it's not that difficult. Basically, there are carbohydrates that you can digest (sugars/starches) and the ones you cannot (fiber). (We'll look at fiber in an upcoming section.)

The carbohydrates that you can digest are fuel for the body. Ultimately they get broken down into either glucose or fructose. Any excess of these two sugars in your diet causes you to manufacture fat either in the liver or your fat tissues because the body can only store limited amounts of sugar as sugar.

Glucose is the master sugar. This is our primary fuel source (along with fat), and every cell in our body can "burn" it to release energy to run the machinery of life.

Digestible starches are made of long-branching pearl necklaces of glucose units. When you eat starch, special chemicals called digestive enzymes cut the string between the pearls. These enzymes called amylases are found in your mouth and your intestine. Their job is to release glucose units from starch so that the body can absorb them.

Unlike glucose, fructose is mainly metabolized in the liver and is primarily turned into fat. This is a key reason why sugary drinks and products high in fructose are so fattening. Alcohol is broken down by the same pathway. The outcome of ingesting too much of either is a fatty liver. This is now the leading cause of liver disease in the US and UK. The damaging by-products can cause inflammation and the end point for some, cirrhosis and liver failure. Dietary fatty liver, so called nonalcohol fatty liver disease (NAFLD) is about to surpass alcohol as the number-one cause of liver transplants in the US!

When you average out sugar consumption in the US, it adds up to about *110 pounds of sugar a year*—an outrageous amount; there is no other way to express that.

By comparison, the average American in 1840 consumed six to eight pounds a year. In 1880, it had risen to thirty pounds. By

1900, it was forty pounds. In 1912, it hit fifty pounds, and the first heart attack was reported. From 1922 to 1972, it remained pretty steady at seventy to eighty pounds. Then, high-fructose corn syrup and corn sugars appeared, along with manufactured food. Consumption rose to ninety pounds by 1980 and blew through 120 pounds in 2000.

Since then, it seems to have stabilized, and the average consumption per person has fallen a little, closer to 110 pounds. However, total consumption in the US continues to rise, suggesting that, although those at the top extreme are cutting their intake, those at the bottom or middle ranges are more than compensating for this by eating more. (Note that this is the average; some people are consuming much more than this!)

In 1972, corn sweeteners, such as high-fructose corn syrups, accounted for less than five pounds of the average American's consumption per year. In 2000, this had reached fifty pounds per year, or nearly half of an average person's consumption. Remember, fructose is turned into fat.

Most individuals living a traditional hunter-gatherer lifestyle consume less than one pound of sugar per year. Like it or not, sugar is directly connected to the current epidemic of obesity and ill health in the US, UK, and around the world.

One of the key take-home messages of this book is that you need to get your sugar consumption under control!

This means going back to eating about twenty to thirty pounds per year. One ounce of sugar equals 6.8 teaspoons, so we are talking about six to ten teaspoons (or cubes) of added sugar per day. This is currently considered to be the maximum safe dose.

So what does that mean in real terms? Would you sit down and eat eight to fifteen cubes of sugar on a plate? No! But here are the figures for some common foods:

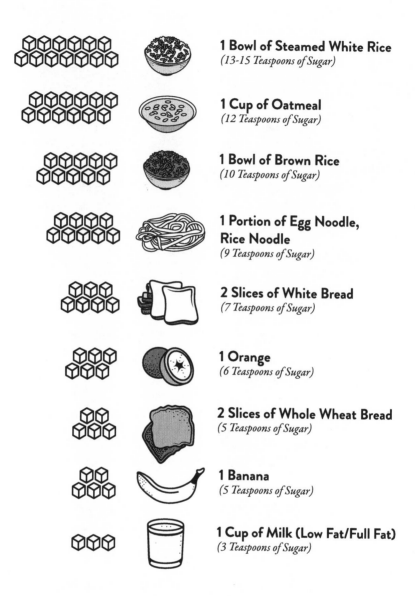

1 Bowl of Steamed White Rice
(13-15 Teaspoons of Sugar)

1 Cup of Oatmeal
(12 Teaspoons of Sugar)

1 Bowl of Brown Rice
(10 Teaspoons of Sugar)

1 Portion of Egg Noodle, Rice Noodle
(9 Teaspoons of Sugar)

2 Slices of White Bread
(7 Teaspoons of Sugar)

1 Orange
(6 Teaspoons of Sugar)

2 Slices of Whole Wheat Bread
(5 Teaspoons of Sugar)

1 Banana
(5 Teaspoons of Sugar)

1 Cup of Milk (Low Fat/Full Fat)
(3 Teaspoons of Sugar)

What is 110 pounds per year? About thirty-three teaspoons per day. That's three cans of soda or four glasses of juice—or one baked potato for lunch and a plate of pasta for dinner.

1 BOWL, 2 CANS

A BOWL OF RICE (HALF A CUP OF COOKED RICE) HAS MORE THAN TWICE THE CARBOHYDRATE CONTENT OF A CAN OF SOFT DRINK.

(model illustrating the type of blood sugar rise that can occur in individuals)

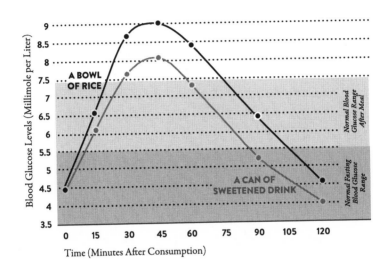

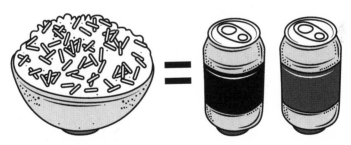

Half a Cup of Cooked Rice

Is Sugar a Drug?

The question of whether sugar is a drug is hotly debated, but I would argue that common sense says it is.

First, watch a baby being given its first taste of sugar. See the expression? Stand by a supermarket checkout line and watch the tantrums as mothers fight their children over the candy rack! Ever been around the

Halloween trick-or-treat experience? Ever watched kids fighting over candies? Do kids trade the very same products? What happens to children when they are fed sugar? Light the blue torch paper, stand back, and watch the fireworks begin. Nice, quiet, "rational" children transform into manic monsters with insane superhuman energy. Wait a little longer and watch the crash. The whining and misery. You may not know much about amphetamine or cocaine, but let me tell you, sugar is the cocaine of childhood. And the reason? It fires up the same circuits in the brain.

Consider your own emotions and experience with sugar. How do you feel when someone suggests that you should stop eating it? Do you relish the idea and feel like celebrating? I don't think so. In fact, in my experience, it is easier to get people off alcohol long term than sugar.

So while the psychologists and researchers debate the question of whether sugar is a drug, the sugar industry and the rest of us follow our evolutionary drives. Why else would food manufacturers add a nutritionally empty substance into 75 percent of their products? Again, it's not rocket science.

> If you don't believe me, google the *National Geographic* article "The Last of the Honey Hunters" and think about the extreme risk and indeed pain that a human will endure to collect this substance.

If you want to be healthy, there is no escaping the facts: you need to cut down your sugar intake. Not a little bit and not even a moderate amount—I mean a lot. In fact, nearly all of it. It has no particular nutritional value. It's just excess energy you don't need, and it turns into inflammation-causing fat. Excessive consumption of glucose causes acute inflammation!

But of course it's not quite that simple. In the UK, sugar consumption and calories have actually gone down slightly while weight continues to go up. We need to look at starch as well.

STARCH

Starch, as previously mentioned, is simply long chains of glucose molecules linked together. This is how plants store the glucose that they make from photosynthesis. Where is it stored? In seeds and tubers—in your food, in grains like rice, wheat, and corn, and of course, potatoes. Indeed most flour from all sources contains starch. This is where the hidden glucose enters our diet.

STARCH

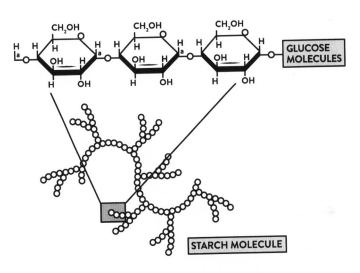

A starch unit is a branching pearl necklace of glucose units.

STARCHY FOODS = SUGAR

In the UK, 20 percent to 25 percent of calories come from wheat-based products, including bread, pizzas, pasta, cakes, and biscuits. In a country with a population of around sixty-four million people, approximately twelve million loaves of bread, ten million cakes and biscuits, and two million pizzas are baked every day.

The average UK consumer takes in 132 pounds (60 kg) of wheat products per year, representing the equivalent of thirty-one cubes of sugar per day. Bread consumption is down, but pizza and pasta more than make up the difference. In comparison, potato consumption is around 170 pounds (77 kg) per year and has been falling steadily for a decade or more. This represents about 1.3 potatoes, equivalent to eleven to twenty cubes of sugar per day.

Combined, this adds up quickly to a total of an equivalent to forty-two cubes of sugar a day! There are sixteen calories in a sugar cube. So this means 670 thermodynamic calories per day in starches. A pound of human fat is 3,500 thermodynamic calories, so it's a fifth of a pound of fat. This is in addition to actual sugar! This is very simplistic but gives you an idea of the scale of the problem and the cause of the current obesity pandemic.

The conclusion you can draw from this is quite straightforward. We all know that too much sugar is bad for you. What most people don't recognize is that starch is actually sugar in another form, and we consume a great deal of it. Most of that consumption is hidden in many of the processed foods we eat, including baked goods. These small amounts all add up to a lot more than you realize.

So here we have it. The Standard American Diet and Standard UK Diet—full of sugar, along with refined and starchy carbohydrates based around wheat, corn, potatoes, and to a lesser extent rice, along with excess added sugars in processed food and drinks—is the primary cause of the current health crisis. Your own health crisis.

Instead of eating sugars and starches, there's a better place to look: foods that are high in fiber.

FIBER: THE KEY TO A HEALTHY GUT AND, IN TURN, YOU

I told you that there are both digestible carbs (sugars and digestible starches), and nondigestible carbs (fibers or resistant starches). As humans, we lack the enzymes to break down this second category, but they are still necessary in our diet.

They serve several functions in plants, but in us they are the primary food for the "healthy" bacteria in our gut. Their digestion by these bacteria produces anti-inflammatory molecules called short-chain fatty acids, or SCFAs for short. This type of starch also slows the digestion and absorption of glucose produced from digestible starch and appears to decrease appetite.

These indigestible starches or fibers get their own mention here because they are one of the key and necessary components of a healthy diet.

Fiber is the common name for the scaffold of plants. It's the stuff that holds them together and gives them structure—the skeleton if you wish. Different parts of the plant have different fibers, and just like everything else involved in diet, some fibers are more beneficial than others.

Roughly, you can divide fiber into two types: soluble (dissolves in water) and insoluble (does not dissolve in water).

Soluble fiber is the best food for your bacterial colony in the large intestine. It comes in substantial quantities in foods like old-fashioned oats. Not only does it hold water in the intestine, but it bulks up the stool and increases the speed that the contents of the gut move along. It can be a great laxative. It also helps lower your cholesterol by decreasing the absorption of bile acids, which are made from cholesterol in the liver. The result is that your body has to use cholesterol to make more bile acids. The net effect is that you dump cholesterol out of the system. This is the reason why oats and other foods high in soluble fiber lower your cholesterol.

Bran is an example of an insoluble fiber. It bulks up feces because it's not broken down by either our own or bacterial enzymes, making them softer and much easier for the intestine to move along, preventing constipation.

To be healthy, you need to consume about thirty-five to forty grams of fiber per day, and you can only get this from plants. This should preferably be in a 50:50 mix of soluble and insoluble.

So what does this look like on a plate? There are about 5.5 grams of fiber in a medium-sized pear, three grams in a cup of strawberries, ten grams in a cup of guacamole or avocado, 4.5 grams in an apple, and three grams in a banana.

Plants tend to contain both types, so you don't need to worry about the soluble-insoluble ratio. I have created a short list below to show how often it's close to a 50:50 mix. (There are lots of charts on the internet if you want more details.)

- Apple with skin: 4.5 grams; 2 grams soluble, 2.5 grams insoluble

- Apricot (1 cup): 4 grams; 2 grams soluble, 2 grams insoluble

- Avocado: 10 grams; 6 grams soluble, 4 grams insoluble

- Oatmeal (1 dry cup): 10 grams; 5 grams soluble, 5 grams insoluble

But the heavy hitters are:

- Kidney beans (1 cup): 12 grams

- Lentils (1 cup): 13 grams

- Split peas (1 cup): 16 grams

- Chickpeas (1 cup): 12 grams

And, believe it or not:

- Dark chocolate: 10 grams per 1 ounce piece.

The bottom line is all plants contain a lot of fiber. The proportions of soluble and insoluble vary a bit, but you need both. Don't get bogged down in the details. Just eat lots of plants in your daily intake of food.

There is no fiber in animal products, such as meat, dairy, eggs, or fish. It does exist as chitin in the exoskeletons of shellfish and insects. Cricket flour has reasonable levels. Realistically, in most modern western diets, it is found only in plant-based foods.

Importantly, you don't find fiber in junk food or the majority of refined or processed foods because it has been removed, and that's dietary madness. In contrast to the brown stuff, white flours, wheat, corn, grits, and white rice are essentially fiber-free.

> The lack of fiber in the modern diet is a significant problem and very much part of the ongoing alterations in the population's gut health and, thus, general health.

Fiber and Your Gut

In simple terms, decreased fiber leads to decreased bacterial production of SCFAs in the gut. These SCFAs—in particular butyrate—are the food that supports the cells that line our intestine, keeping the intestine wall healthy and functioning normally, helping maintain its barrier function. No- or low-fiber diets translate into low butyrate and an unhappy gut.

Not only does butyrate keep the lining of the intestine healthy and working as a dynamically controlled border, but it also causes an active decrease in the amount of inflammation by modulating the activity of the neuro-immune system lining the gut wall. This anti-inflammatory effect is not confined to the intestine due to the gut neuro-immune network's impact on the entire body.

Butyrate and other SCFAs also lower cholesterol by inhibiting its storage in liver cells. So fiber has a double cholesterol-lowering role by removing cholesterol from the body, as discussed in the previous section, *and* decreasing its formation in liver cells.

Last on the fiber topic, when sugars and starches are eaten in their natural form, mixed with lots of fiber as in fruits and vegetables, the rate at which the body breaks down the food is slowed. This translates into a decreased rate of absorption of the sugars produced by digestion, providing for a low glycemic index. Rapid absorption causes high spikes of blood glucose, which in turn causes surges in your insulin levels, creating all sorts of negative issues for your metabolism. This is why you should eat minimally processed grains. And gluten-free flours have the same effect; they are starch rich, just no wheat in them.

Brown versus white rice and whole-grain versus white breads contain a similar amount of starch, so they have the same *glycemic load*. But because the "brown versions" are packaged with the fiber in their coverings, they slow the sugar spike while contributing to your total insoluble fiber intake as well. Thus, they have a low *glycemic index*.

All these things are key reasons why you need to significantly increase your vegetable and fruit consumption, aiming for at least thirty-five grams of fiber per day.

My own go-to for all my patients, and indeed myself, is Dr. Sam's porridge oats breakfast! A cup of old-fashioned oatmeal porridge cooked in water with a banana, a chopped-up apple, a handful of blueberries, and some ground flaxseed, all topped off with some real, as in live, yogurt.

This is bacteria breakfast as much as it is breakfast for you. For those who struggle with veggies, try this every day for a month, and you will be surprised at what happens to your bathroom habits and general health.

GLYCEMIC INDEX AND GLYCEMIC LOAD OF POPULAR FOODS

■ Low ■ Medium □ High

TYPE OF FOOD	GLYCEMIC INDEX	SERVING SIZE	NET CARBS	GLYCEMIC LOAD
Glucose	100	(50g)	50	50
Snickers Bar	55	1 bar (113g)	64	35
White Rice	64	1 cup (186g)	52	33
Potato Chips	54	4 oz (114g)	55	30
Macaroni and Cheese	64	1 serving (166g)	47	30
Baked Potato	85	1 medium (173g)	33	28
Brown Rice	55	1 cup (195g)	42	23
Raisins	64	1 small box (43g)	32	20
Spaghetti	42	1 cup (140g)	38	16
Low-Fat Yogurt	33	1 cup (245g)	47	16
Bananas	52	1 large (136g)	27	14
Pizza	30	2 slices (260g)	42	13
Oatmeal	58	1 cup (234g)	21	12
White Bread	70	1 slice (30g)	14	10
Ice Cream	61	1 cup (72g)	16	10
Honey	55	1 tbsp (21g)	17	9
Sugar (Sucrose)	68	1 tbsp (12g)	12	8
Watermelon	72	1 cup (154g)	11	8
Popcorn	72	2 cup (16g)	10	7
Apples	38	1 medium (138g)	16	6
Oranges	48	1 medium (131g)	12	6
Grapefruit	25	1/2 large (166g)	11	3
Peanuts	14	4 oz (113g)	15	2
Carrots	47	1 large (72g)	5	2
Bean Sprouts	25	1 cup (104g)	4	1

A BRIEF MENTION OF SALT

The idea that almost all of us should be cutting back on our salt intake to avoid high blood pressure is well-entrenched in both the general population and physicians' minds. But how strong is the evidence for this view? The simple answer is that it is weak. Unfortunately, salt restriction is now so much a part of conventional wisdom, in a way that goes beyond the evidence, that it is hard to know where to get reliable advice about it.

The issue, of course, arises due to the use of salt in manufactured foods and to some extent in restaurant food. Every cook knows that adding a little salt (seasoning) spices up the taste.

But as long as you are avoiding processed and junk food, you do not need to worry about salt.

Of course, you should worry about high blood pressure. Equally, or arguably more important than taking blood pressure medication is avoiding processed food with its high sugar and salt content, along with losing weight, doing some type of exercise, and getting proper rest (topics for Chapters 4 and 5!). These will do as much to reduce your blood pressure as cutting back on salt.

Indeed, if you are on a healthy real-food diet, you need to *add* some salt. I regularly see individuals who eat well but become salt- and thus water-depleted. This leads to low blood pressure and a myriad of unpleasant symptoms, such as fatigue, weakness, and muscle cramps.

So the name of the game is real foods, mainly plants, not too much, and a little bit of added salt.

What to Eat

I promised you that after focusing on what *not* to eat (or at least what to eat less of), we would talk about what *to* eat. So here is your basic guide.

You should strive to eat:

- Eighty percent **veggies** and **fruit** (80 percent veggies/20 percent fruit), **(VF)**

- Ten percent **animal** products: meats, eggs, dairy, cheeses (modest), seafood **(A)**

- Ten percent **grains**: rice/wheat (bread and pasta)/corn/grits, quinoa, rye **(G)**

As a basic guide, I've broken it down to what you can eat freely, what you should eat in moderation, what you can eat occasionally, and what you should eat only rarely. There is no meal plan for a good reason. I don't know what you eat, or more importantly what you like to eat. Lots of people buy books and meal plans and struggle to stick to them because they're not the foods they enjoy. Most of us have six to eight standard go-to meals, and that's fine. Just modify them to meet these proportions and adjust the quantity on the plate. Remember, not too much! That way you can plan your diet around what you like to eat.

So no exact portions. You just need a guide. Honestly, if you cut back the sugar and starches and increase your vegetables, it will all sort itself out.

MAY EAT FREELY

- All vegetables, especially green leafy vegetables. Think of a rainbow of colors **(VF)**

- Nuts (cashews, almonds, walnuts, pistachios, macadamias, etc.) **(VF)**

- Seeds (sunflower seeds, pumpkin seeds, chia seeds, hemp seeds) **(VF)**

MAY EAT MODERATELY

- Fruit (three servings per day) **(VF)**

  - Lower sugar: all berries, apples, pears, kiwis, oranges, watermelon, and cantaloupe (Best choice)

  - Higher sugar: pineapple, mangoes, bananas, grapes

- Chicken **(A)**

- Fish **(A)**

- Seafood **(A)**

- Lamb **(A)**

- Salad dressings (best is olive oil and vinegar) **(VF)**

- Cheese and other dairy products **(A)**

- Eggs **(A)**

- Grains, such as brown rice, oats, quinoa, spelt, amaranth, chickpea flour, millet **(G)**

MAY EAT OCCASIONALLY (ONE TO TWO SERVINGS PER WEEK)

- Red meats **(A)**

- Pork **(A)**

RARELY EAT (TWO TO FOUR PER MONTH)

- Added refined sugar (including syrups and packaged goods with sugar)

- Packaged and processed foods (most contain hidden sugar)

- Juice (all contain a great deal of sugar—six teaspoons in a typical juice box)

- Soda (eight to ten teaspoons sugar per can)

- Sports drinks

- Bread (wheat flour = sugar)

- Pasta (wheat flour = sugar)

- Cream of wheat (wheat flour = sugar)

- Grits (corn = sugar)

- Potatoes (potato = sugar)

- Baked goods (biscuits/cookies and cakes. Wheat flour = sugar)

- Rice (rice = sugar)

Carbs (and fats) are fuel. So if your tummy size and weight are appropriate, and you are exercising, then you can add back more carbs.

FATS

The best source of fats is generally plants, olives, olive oil, avocados, and nuts. But modest amounts of butter (not margarine), eggs, and dairy are fine. Oily fish are also excellent sources. Sadly, mercury levels in fish are beginning to make this less safe. Sardines and anchovies are perhaps the best as they are low on the food chain.

PROTEIN

Mix it up from plant and animal sources. Keep it simple: the goal is around 0.75–1.0 grams per kilogram body weight. For the average person, that's around fifty to seventy grams per day—which is three to four fillets of fish, three tins of sardines, or one large chicken breast. As you age, you need to be on the higher end of the protein intake scale, but be careful not to overdo it—too much protein, just like too much sugar, is inflammatory.

WATER

Water intake and adequate hydration are critical to health and normal body and brain function. There is a lot of confusing advice about this topic, and I take the following approach. Your state of hydration is easily assessed by the color and the quantity of urine you produce. The goal is urine that looks like a glass of water or very diluted yellow lemonade. In regards to quantity, at least five to six urinations per day. So don't fret too much about the six to eight glass rule; just monitor your bathroom habits and urine color, aiming for the above. Thirst only occurs when you are already significantly dehydrated, and in older individuals, this feeling is blunted, which means that as you age, it is critical that you are actively mindful of your water intake.

VITAMINS AND SUPPLEMENTS

We pay a lot of attention to the so-called macronutrients—carbohy-drates, fat, and protein—and this of course is important. However, there are many minerals, vitamins, and micronutrients that the body requires to function properly. Some of these are easily obtained from pretty much any diet, and some are not.

As a general comment, a balanced diet of 80 percent vegetables and fruit, 10 percent grains, and 10 percent animal products should provide all the nutrients that you need.

This diet is best with variety in your choice of different vegetables and fruit. I would suggest the same for grain, staying away from wheat and corn and experimenting with other types of whole grains. In re-gards to animal products, return to using the entire animal, not just the flesh. In particular, the liver, in naturally fed, grass-raised animals, is a nutrient-rich source of many important vitamins. However, if the animal was not reared properly, the liver is the clearing house of drugs and hormones used in factory farming.

Aside from food, especially plant-based foods, minerals and trace minerals come from our water supplies. The content varies depending on where you live. As part of our ongoing poisoning of our environment through poor farming practices forced upon farmers, and chemicals from industry escaping or being released in an indiscriminate manner, most of our ground and river water is no longer safe to drink. The response is that we have turned to purified and bottled water. It may be true that this water is safe in the sense that it is free from most toxins, excluding the fact that it is stored in plastic bottles. However, it is also devoid of the minerals and trace elements essential for a healthy body.

The net result I recommend is a multivitamin with minerals a couple of times per week.

Vitamins are chemicals, or more correctly molecules, that are critical components to many of our chemical or metabolic processes. We give them a special category because we are unable to make them in the body, and so we need them in our food. Out of the many hundreds, here are four critical ones I have chosen to highlight.

- Vitamin D is crucial to health. It is one of the oldest biological compounds on the planet and probably played a role in single cells joining together to make multicellular organisms like us. It is not really a vitamin, as we are supposed to make it in our skin from sun exposure. It is really a hormone. Given how long it has existed, it's no wonder it is so critical to health. It influences over 1,000 human genes in the body, which means it influences around 4 percent of our genetic code. Most of these genes are related to immune system function (housekeeping), but vitamin D receptors are also found in the part of the brain regulating sleep, along with other sites in the central nervous system. Vitamin D also seems to have an influence on the composition of the gut microbiota. Because we typically stay indoors or are covered up when we go outside, most people are deficient and need to take a supplement. A range of about 1,000–4,000 IU per day is a safe dose. Of course some sunshine on your skin would be best.

- Vitamin K2, or menaquinone, is critical for bone, gum, and blood vessel health. Most have never even heard of it. Main sources were grass-fed animal liver, which we no longer eat, and some dairy products. Swiss mountain farmers have known this for centuries and give the first spring butter to the elderly and pregnant mothers. The Japanese get it from natto, a fermented soy product. I recommend this supplement to everyone; 70–140 micrograms a day is fine.

- The B vitamins are a diverse group of molecules that our bodies need to manage; they perform a multitude of chemical processes that keep us alive and healthy. They are present in food in varying amounts, but there is an increasing body of evidence that yet again the intestinal microbiota is key. It would appear that specialist species within the gut not only make these vitamins for the rest of the colony but are also producing them for us.

- Magnesium is a key mineral, and yet 70 percent or more of people fail to reach their required daily intake. It is the hemoglobin of plants. Iron is what we use to make hemoglobin. It's the protein that carries oxygen around our body. Magnesium is at the core of chlorophyll; it's the substance that makes plants green and makes glucose from sunlight. This failure to get enough magnesium reflects the lack of intake of green leafy plants. Magnesium plays several critical roles in human metabolism.

A quick connection between sleep, microbiota, and nutrition: We now know that along with diet and vitamin D, the B vitamins can influence the composition of the colony, and, in turn, the colony composition is important in regards to the production of vitamins. Vitamins D and B5 (pantothenic acid) have an influence on the regions of the brain that control both the quantity and the architecture of sleep. Low vitamin D and possibly pantothenic acid, along with other Bs, affect the quality of our sleep. If you are sleeping badly, restoring vitamin D levels along with judicious use of B supplements can improve sleep patterns in many patients.

When to Eat

How and when you eat matters.

The way we eat and digest food is a very complex process requiring a coordinated interaction among several body systems. Understanding this requires a little dip into how the body works again.

The central nervous system—our brain and spinal cord—connects to the peripheral nervous system and the enteric nervous system that are found in the gut wall. There is also the autonomic system that controls body functions. This itself is divided into two parts.

The *sympathetic* branch controls all things associated with not being at rest. This system is closely associated with adrenaline (epinephrine) and a neurotransmitter called noradrenalin (norepinephrine); it's also called the fight-or-flight system. The sympathetic state occurs when running around, being busy, exercising, or being stressed, and it shuts down normal digestion.

The other half of the autonomic system is the *parasympathetic* system. It drives the rest-and-digest body state.

The two systems should be in balance. But the sympathetic system is often dominant in our hectic, high-stress, modern lifestyles.

We need to eat when we can rest and digest. When the parasympathetic system is favored, the processes of eating and digestion can work normally. But if you are in sympathetic mode, then the digestive process can go awry. That can create a whole host of intestinal issues, including IBS.

This is important, as it dictates when you should be eating. If you eat on the run, so to speak, you are setting yourself up for improper digestion.

Acid reflux is one of the most common digestive diseases affecting 20 percent of the population—and in some, it's associated with autonomic nervous system imbalance. Eating quickly or when on the go means more sympathetic and less parasympathetic activity.

Typically the body goes through a four-stage cycle from eating to finishing digestion. This takes several hours, and then the gut cleans itself. It literally washes itself.

So timing when you eat matters! In practical terms, I tell patients that if you cannot eat and then sit still for sixty minutes, you might consider skipping that meal (a good opportunity to practice "intermittent fasting"). Certainly, you should not eat more frequently than every four hours, so cut the snacks however small, and a minimum of twelve hours without food overnight.

Your To-Do List

- Listen to Michael Pollan, and "eat real food, mainly plants, and not a lot."

- Follow 80/10/10: eat 80 percent vegetables and fruit, 10 percent animal products, 10 percent grains

- Consume thirty-five to forty grams of fiber per day.

- Eat fifty to seventy grams of protein from plant or animal sources per day.

- Eat less

    - Stop snacking

    - Consider eating only one or two meals per day. You'll be fine.

    - Skip meals (now called intermittent fasting) at least a few days per week.

- Avoid junk food like you avoid poison.

- Quit sugar except on special days. No more than three to six teaspoons of added sugar per day!

    - Stop drinking all sodas and juices. It's seven to ten teaspoons of sugar per serving!

    - Read food labels. It's scary how much sugar is added and what else is in there.

    - If you do eat food from a box or packets, as a general rule, if you cannot pronounce the name of any ingredient on the label, or if there are more than two added ingredients that you don't recognize, avoid the product.

    - Decrease your refined starches (white flours from any source, rice, pasta, and potatoes). They are sugar in another form and drive high cholesterol levels and fatty tissue production along with chronic inflammation.

- Keep grains and grain-based foods at or below 10 percent of your daily diet. They are primarily starches.

- Use supplements intelligently. Consider adding microminerals, vitamin D3, and K2, along with the B vitamins and definitely B12 if you are truly vegan.

- Make sure that your animal product consumption includes organ meats from grass-fed animals as well as fish.

- Feed your gut microbes, such as Dr. Sam's microbiota porridge oats breakfast! A cup of old-fashioned oatmeal porridge cooked in water with a banana, a chopped up apple, a handful of blueberries, and some freshly ground flaxseed. Top it off with real live yogurt.

Your diet is the primary ingredient in your health. It is arguable that diet is the single most important cultural change that has led to our current health crises. The other issues we will cover next—exercise, sleep, Me-Time, and stress reduction—are important, but diet is *critical*.

This chapter contains a great deal of information, but that's the point. To make helpful choices, people need information, and that is what I have attempted to provide. It was long, but you are now armed with *all* the essential knowledge. Any more is too much and falls into the realm of therapeutics or metabolic hacking.

But, as crucial as your diet is, it's only the first of our Five Elements. Now, it's time to get moving! Chapter 4 is about exercise.

CHAPTER 4

ESSENTIAL EXERCISE

· ·

Until the very recent past, physical activity was simply part of everyday life. Before the era of mechanization, everything—and I mean everything—required you to use your body. In that sense, exercise was hidden and emotionally effortless.

Over the last few decades, physical activity in the population has decreased dramatically. We drive to work or ride the bus, sit at work, ride or drive home, and then watch TV or play video games.

A wonderfully clever piece of research, conducted in the days when London buses had both drivers and conductors, showed that the drivers had significantly worse health parameters, decreased longevity, and healthspans, despite coming from the same backgrounds and subjected to the same environment. The only difference was the sedentary nature of the drivers' work. Indeed the conductors had a higher stress job dealing with the passengers.

The Benefits of Exercise

In the modern world, our lives have become predominantly sedentary. Exercise is no longer effortless for most, and it has become a separate activity that requires that we make space in our day to do it.

Regular exercise is not an optional extra.

But a sedentary lifestyle is a health disaster. Sitting in an office all day is probably equivalent to smoking a pack of cigarettes. Being sedentary is a recipe for early death and increased levels of illness. Taking some exercise has the opposite effect.

The benefits of daily exercise and movement far surpass any amount of medication or medical intervention, and even modest amounts at any age can produce positive results. No medicine in any pharmacy gets even close to reducing the risk of disease. If you survive your first heart attack, we have known for decades that just going for a short daily walk significantly decreases your chance of a second one compared to someone who remains sedentary. There is probably no single medical condition that cannot be improved by exercise, impacting both physical and mental well-being.

Just as diet is medicine, so is exercise. We all know this, so while many of us find it uncomfortable and tedious, we all recognize that we feel uplifted and so much better after we have done it. It's the doing that is the challenge, not the post-exercise feeling of wellness. If you are struggling, focus on how good you feel afterwards and mentally downplay the uncomfortable doing part. (This is an excellent example of being mindful, which we will explore in a later chapter.)

EXERCISE AND INFLAMMATION

We've known for a long time that a predominantly sedentary lifestyle significantly increases the risk of just about any disease you can imagine. This includes both infectious diseases and inflammation-based, chronic, noncommunicable diseases. Type 2 diabetes and high blood pressure, blood vessel disease (atheroma), heart disease, lung diseases like COPD, cancers, depression, and dementia are much more common in people who don't take any exercise.

One of the reasons this occurs is because physical inactivity promotes the buildup of intra-abdominal fat. This type of fat, also known as visceral fat, leads to inflammation in the body for two reasons. The first is that fat cells themselves produce inflammatory molecules (adipokines) that enter the bloodstream and circulate the entire body. The second is, for reasons that we don't understand, type-one macrophages (M1 macrophages), an important immune system cell that accumulates in visceral fat and secretes a steady stream of inflammatory molecules. The effect is the promotion of body-wide, chronic, low-grade background inflammation.

. . . .

A large tummy equals increased inflammation.

. . . .

Exercise decreases intra-abdominal fat, even in the absence of weight loss. If you exercise regularly, you change the proportion of "bad" abdominal fat for healthier peripheral fat. This is one reason I suggest that people don't get fixated on their scale. They are better off having a relationship with a tape measure. As we established in Chapter 3, measuring your tummy size is a much more helpful metric of health than weight.

We know that chronic inflammation is an essential part of accelerating the aging process, along with the initiation and progression of a broad range of age-related illnesses and diseases. Physical exercise helps prevent these conditions, and one of the links has now been found. If you measure the anti-inflammatory marker IL-10 in the blood, there is a significant increase following exercise, thus making exercise itself an anti-inflammatory process.

Contracting muscles also release the chemical IL-6 into the circulation, which in turn activates several beneficial networks. Interestingly, this cytokine, which often plays an inflammatory role when released from exercising muscles, works in quite the opposite fashion, causing a significant decrease in the activity of several parts of the immune system, damping down inflammation. You can overdo it, and it is long recognized that extreme exercise can be associated with increased risks of infections and possibly cancer. This might occur because of actual immunosuppression in very fit and active athletes caused by these IL-6 and IL-10 pathways, along with others that we have yet to work out.

We don't know where the balance lies in the contribution made by visceral fat and that made by contracting muscles. Suffice to say, regular and moderate exercise coupled with trimming down your intra-abdominal fat leads to measurable decreases in inflammatory markers and inflammation throughout the body. That's an excellent thing.

EXERCISE AND THE BRAIN

All of us know somebody with dementia or Alzheimer's disease, and I recognize that a lot of my middle-aged patients worry about it, wondering, *Will it happen to me?*

The straightforward answer is that it could. We are beginning to understand the processes behind early dementia and Alzheimer's disease. Again, we run into our old enemy: chronic inflammation. Just as this process damages joints and blood vessels, it can also harm the brain.

Because inflammation is so important, it is covered in detail in several parts of this book, so here we'll focus on the data supporting the beneficial effects of exercise on the brain.

The good news is there are ways of protecting yourself. The information coming out of current scientific research clearly shows that exercise has a significant impact on your brain and cognitive health.

We can demonstrate clear and remarkable benefits on learning abilities, memory, and evidence of protection from neurodegenerative diseases. Interestingly, there is also strong evidence showing that exercise is just as effective for treating depression as taking an antidepressant.

The changes that we see in the central nervous system are very real in a practical sense. They include an enhanced ability to learn and improvements in not only memory but also problem-solving skills.

They are also structural, with a delay in the loss of actual brain substance, particularly in areas that we use for thinking. When neuroscientists look at brain structures in those who exercise, they find an increased ability to form new nerve cells and increased connections between nerve cells. They also notice an increase in the number of blood vessels, which improves the amount of oxygen and nutrients reaching those cells.

Lastly, exercise actually causes a central suppression of your appetite. So far from wanting to eat more after exercising, you actually feel less hungry!

METABOLIC FLEXIBILITY AND EXERCISE

One of the great benefits of taking some exercise and moving is that it improves metabolic flexibility. The body has two main fuel choices to create the energy required to run the machinery of life: glucose (carb fuel) or ketones (fat fuel). Metabolic flexibility is the ability of the body to switch from one type of fuel to the other.

If you are sedentary, the body can find it challenging to make the switch. Here's why: natural processes in living organisms are, on the whole, efficient. If the body is forced to use a particular pathway to do something, it builds the machinery to do that and tears down the machinery it is not operating. So if you do not burn fat regularly, the body loses the ability to do so.

We are not sure why, but when you exercise regularly, the body maintains the machinery required to utilize both fuel types, meaning that it is equally happy burning glucose or ketones. This is metabolic flexibility. That can only be good news if you need to burn fat.

In contrast, physical inactivity and sedentary behaviors lead to metabolic inflexibility. Your body gets stuck in carb-burning metabolism. Not only does it not burn fat, but after a while, it *cannot* burn fat, and so you find it hard to lose your fat stores.

Exercise leads to the production of adiponectin by the fat tissue cells. This is one of the main hormones that causes the fat stores to break down fat to ketones and export it for fuel.

. . . .

Although exercise is the wrong way to lose weight in terms of simply burning calories (a one-hour brisk walk burns 400 calories—that's a cheese and mayo sandwich), exercise does promote the burning of fat stores for fuel and the redistribution of dangerous intra-abdominal or visceral fat to other parts of the body.

. . . .

EXERCISE AND CANCER

There is an increasing body of evidence that clearly supports the idea that exercise has an impact on the natural history of cancer. The effect is an improvement in the quality of life for many patients, and indeed it appears to also increase length of survival in some. There is better tolerance of cancer therapies and possibly improved responses to therapy.

Here is an area where yoga comes into its own, and I personally believe that all cancer patients should be taught essential yoga based around breathing and basic movements.

If you are well enough, add some form of impact activity—for example using a step or skipping. There seem to be gains over simple aerobic and strength-based protocols, particularly in the area of maintaining strong bones.

POSTURE

Posture may seem like a strange topic to find in the chapter on exercise, but it is critical to good health. This is why osteopaths and chiropractors have such strong followings. These two healing disciplines deal with balance, in particular muscle balance, and their founders understood the importance of being in equilibrium and indeed the connection between this and overall well-being of body and mind.

There is no doubt that developing core strength, flexibility, and good posture has a profound effect on your physical health—and by that I mean it affects every system in the body.

Most interesting to me is that it affects your mental well-being as well. Standing up straight improves your mood and your cognitive function. The converse is also true: if you slouch or tend to be hunched up in your posture, you need to do something about it. Go see a physiotherapist, chiropractor, osteopath, or indeed a good and educated personal trainer and get some help in improving how you sit, stand, and hold yourself.

So be mindful and pay attention to your posture. If you are struggling emotionally, force yourself to stand up straight. If you really want to go for it, throw your arms above your head in a victory pose. Try it and see what happens.

EMOTIONS ARE PHYSICAL EVENTS

As you begin to address your health challenges, it's important that you understand that emotions are physical events. They do not occur in your mind alone; they occur throughout the whole body. We all recognize this but perhaps fail to understand the importance of this statement.

When you experience an emotion, there is always a whole-body physical change. Everyone has had a "near miss" or had a bit of terrible news. Think about how you felt. Cold chills, shivers down your spine, that all-over body flush, for some if the news is really bad, vomiting or even collapse.

If you are happy, you feel light and bouncy; you stand tall, and your facial expressions change. All of this is automatic and occurs unconsciously. Sadness and depression produce a heavy feeling in the body, so you slouch, and your facial expressions broadcast your mood. Our ability to exercise and our muscle strength is reduced, and we fatigue more easily.

Interestingly, you can create emotions by acting out the body posture. This is a crucial piece of information because you can use this to alter your emotional state by changing your physical posture and facial expressions. Force yourself to sit up straight and smile. You will feel better. Take a victory stance and your whole body and mind is altered in a positive fashion. Sound odd? Well maybe, but it's a psychological fact.

Try this fun trick: raise your eyebrows and then try to say something angry or mean. It's difficult and indeed impossible to be convincing. Now crunch them together and try again. Easy. Keep them crunched and try to say something loving or kind. Again, it does not work.

Posture and facial expressions matter because they have a profound effect on your neuro-immune system.

We use these techniques in therapy to break certain mind and emotional states. When you are angry or locked in fright, flight, or freeze mode of sympathetic overdrive for whatever reason, you cannot learn or comprehend. As therapists, we cannot connect with you; your frontal lobes and amygdala go offline, and what we say or do has absolutely no effect toward helping you. Eye movement desensitization reprogramming (EMDR) represents this perfectly. When individuals are overwhelmed, as in the treatment of post-traumatic stress disorder, therapists can unlock the frontal cortex and emotional processing centers in the midbrain by simply using eye movements. This then allows the patient to come out of the freeze state and process the emotions and therapist's training.

Now that you are aware of the benefits of exercise, let's look at how you can exercise more effectively so you can take advantage of all those health benefits.

How to Exercise Effectively

The goal of exercise is to maintain functional and mental fitness, and reduce body-wide background inflammation.

As we age, most people lose strength, coordination, and balance. They simply cannot do the things they want to do. When you choose an exercise program, remember that it must benefit you. It has to have *functional gains*: effects that allow you to live the life you want to live and do the things you enjoy, all the way into old age. Here is how to do it.

It's true that the majority of us find exercise a challenge, but it doesn't have to be. Try introducing it wherever you can. Yes, you've heard it before: use the stairs, not the elevator, cycle to the gym rather than driving your car, and so on. Reintroduce little bits of exercise and movement wherever you can as part of your day. Most of us don't live in a country with easy access to lovely walks or hikes, but that doesn't stop you from walking to the park or the shops down the road.

· ·

All school kids should have exercise as part of their working day. The data is clear and robust: fifteen minutes of low-impact morning PE (as I experienced each day after assembly and before lessons) has a profound impact on the quality of learning. Couple this with a later start time and an hour of extra sleep, and school grades would go up in a way politicians and educators can only dream of.

· ·

There is a dose-dependent relationship between the amount of exercise and the beneficial effects. You'll be happy to hear that moderate exercise is the most helpful. So don't worry if you don't enjoy it. Walking is more than sufficient—that is, if you walk far enough.

In the rest of this chapter, we'll take a look at some different forms of exercise so you can build your plan. But remember: You do not need to go to a gym! You need to bring simple exercise to your day-to-day life, and the easiest and very best way to do this is by walking.

WALKING

Good news for those who struggle with exercise. There is a simple solution: walk. Humans were designed and evolved to walk. It was our mode of transport since our ancestors stood up on two feet, moving one in front of the other. We are good at it.

It's impossible to overstate the benefits of just walking as much as you can. The more you do, the better off you will be, both physically and mentally. It's that simple: get out of the car and walk.

Walk upstairs, walk to the store, and walk to work. Walk in the park, who cares where; just do it and you will benefit. And don't believe those who tell you it's not as good as vigorous exercise. Studies show that it's just as beneficial.

How much should you walk? Four miles per day would be a great start. That's an hour at a very brisk pace, and fifteen minutes longer at a slower one. There is no doubt that more is beneficial, and if you can get up to ten miles (20,000 steps) daily, you will likely never be overweight or diabetic!!

There are no downsides to walking. It's what the human body was designed to do.

As with swimming, and unlike many other sports, it's almost impossible to seriously injure yourself walking. Most of us are not natural runners, and indeed many injure themselves doing this activity. Not that we cannot run, and certainly the human body has the capacity to jog or lope very long distances. But if you do run or jog, get someone to teach you and buy some good shoes. The older you are, the more this matters. Now I'm not suggesting people should not run. For many it is an excellent escape from the office and a beneficial form of exercise, but be careful when starting out. In contrast, very few manage to injure themselves walking. Any distance is helpful, even at a slow pace.

CYCLING

Cycling is another absolute winner. I recommend cycling to everyone. It's a non-weight-bearing exercise that, like walking, has utility. It gets you somewhere. The move toward using bicycles in many cities is a tremendous reinvention of this excellent, non-polluting form of transport. Bicycles are one of the most efficient pieces of machinery ever invented by man.

Pretty much anyone and everyone can ride a bike. They come in all different types and sizes depending upon your needs and desires. From sit-up and beg, slow-moving bikes with a basket, to top-notch road or off-road racing bikes, all offer an excellent opportunity to take some cardio and all-important leg-resistance exercise while moving from point A to B.

. . . .

We know that increased strength in leg muscles has greater health benefits than arm strength.

. . . .

SWIMMING

Swimming is also a non-weight-bearing exercise. This takes on enormous importance for so many who suffer from joint problems. It offers an opportunity to move against resistance without the effect of gravity.

Swimming is also one of those all-over body exercises, using every muscle you have. Better still, it's difficult to overdo it, so it's tough to injure yourself. (Not impossible, but difficult.)

When you swim in the pool or outdoors, you develop a meditative rhythm, both in your repetitive movement and your breathing. Rhythmic breathing is the basis of all meditative practices. If you spend thirty to forty minutes with your head in the water, it's Me-Time—just you, alone with your thoughts. (We'll discuss the absolute importance of Me-Time in Chapter 6.)

When I swim, I like to mix it up. Sometimes I concentrate on my technique, focusing my mind on my body and individual muscles.

Other times, I let my body go into auto-mode and watch my mind and its thoughts. True meditation.

Last, there is a vast body of evidence that supports the idea that being beside or in water is just good for you. Why else would we all love to head to the beach or the lake for a break, lounge in a warm bath, or have all our best ideas in the shower? Water is life. Use it whenever you can.

YOGA

Everyone should try yoga or its derivative, pilates! Why? Because, minute for minute, it's an excellent use of your time. Not only are you taking some exercise, but it is also a meditation, an opportunity to get in touch with yourself physically and emotionally.

So many people are put off by yoga because its "trendy"—something that slim twenty-three-year-olds do in tight clothing, which requires flexibility and strength, needs a studio, and is foreign, spiritual, or difficult. The reality is that it is none of the above.

Anyone can practice yoga at any age. You don't have to be fit or flexible. You don't have to be spiritual. It's nothing but good for you.

Yoga is a way of life, and yogis follow a particular philosophy that includes diet, meditation practice based on breath work, and a non-dogmatic, spiritual belief system. But you can simply use the exercise part and the breath work to great health benefit. In reality, this is what most westerners going to studios do.

So why am I so keen on you learning some basic yoga? Because it's another all-over body exercise. It's also an all-over body stretch. Most importantly, it teaches you to pay attention to your physical and mental self. You can do it in a five-to-fifteen-minute session daily, and the benefits of even five minutes are well worth the effort. So if you don't like exercise, this is your best bet regarding a return on your time investment. I promise that if you stick to a daily ten-to-fifteen-minute routine for thirty days, you will notice a significant change.

There is a short learning curve of some basic movements, and you need a mat and a bit of space. There are so many apps and videos that it's easy to find one for you. Choose a simple morning flow routine. Once you are comfortable and have some basics, be brave and go to a beginner's class at a studio. Join a clan.

If you are very unfit or overweight, don't worry. There are still plenty of videos for you. You can even start in a chair. Essential parts of yoga are available to anyone.

The great benefit of yoga both as an exercise and as a breathing practice is that it connects you with your body. It is movement and Me-Time rolled into one. It can all be completed in fifteen minutes.

Consider making it a morning habit or ritual and set yourself up for the day. It's a great transition from sleep to wakefulness, and it's a great time to check in on yourself every morning.

CROSSFIT

I don't necessarily enjoy the competitive nature of CrossFit, but other than that I am a big fan of the style and philosophy behind this ever-expanding movement (religion?). For most of us, exercise only makes sense if it has purpose and real benefit. The fundamental principle behind CrossFit–style training/exercise is that it promotes functionality. Its goal: to allow you to be able to live the life you choose without impediment and enjoy the things you love unhampered by physical decline. As such, it focuses on strength, balance, and coordination. Brilliant! The added gain for me, in spite of my dislike of the competitive aspect, is I love the community concept, which as you will see is critical to overall health and longevity.

TAI CHI

Tai chi has its origins in the east and, like yoga, focuses the mind and the body through a series of rehearsed flowing movements. It is particularly helpful for older individuals and those with limited mobility, but it can be practiced by anyone at any age. It is used as a daily communal or community activity throughout China, other Asian countries, and increasingly around the world. Its significant physical and mental health benefits are scientifically documented. Again, it's an activity bringing people together in a cooperative and supportive environment with a shared goal.

SPORTS

Playing sports has many advantages over exercising alone. On the whole, they are group activities. Even if you partake in individual sports, like solo dinghy sailing or kayaking, there is the important benefit of belonging to a group, a clan. As I keep mentioning, the importance of being part of a group of people cannot be overstated. When we work together in a cooperative fashion, there are significant benefits to your mental health and levels of happiness, and this, as you are learning, translates into better physical health.

SEX

No book on health, wellness, and longevity could be complete without discussing this most essential aspect of human existence: sex.

The reality is that if you are lucky enough to have one, the incorporation of a healthy sex life into your exercise routine is a massive booster of health and well-being. But sex and sexuality are complex.

Different cultures deal with sex in diverse ways, with many unfortunately placing it into some special box: naughty, immoral, or some other negative connotations. But the biological reality is that human touch and warmth is life sustaining. This starts from conception and continues throughout life. In the early days of incubators for premature babies, pediatricians thought that babies need to be sterile. There was a minimal touch policy. Sadly, many babies died, and no one could figure out why. Then someone went against the grain and started holding babies. The effect was astounding. The decrease in mortality was stunning.

This need for physical comfort never leaves us; it's with us from the cradle to the grave. Even holding the hand of a dying person can bring great relief.

Sex is part of this phenomenon. Of course, there is the all-important role of procreation, the making of the next generation. However, this is perhaps the practical role of sex, a fantastic biological function and process, but sex is so much more.

In its most basic form, and the reason it exists, is that physical contact and expression of comforting and sharing with another or others is crucial to our well-being. A handshake, a hug, even just sitting close to another person makes us feel good. It's part of the group- or tribal-bonding process that evolved to keep us safe.

This is not a book about the diversity of sexual expression and sex, but it encompasses so much that it cannot be ignored as a health-boosting activity. It embraces communication, connecting, contribution, and coping—four of the five Cs of happiness, as you will soon learn more about—and it is typically pleasurable. Sexual activity with a trusted partner has immense psychological and physical benefits.

Part of this is the expression by the nervous and the endocrine systems of several feel-good neuro-chemicals. These include dopamine (anticipation of pleasure) and endorphins (elation), along with oxytocin (the cuddle hormone) and prolactin (satisfaction and relaxation).

We know that sex relieves stress and improves the quality of your sleep. It boosts your immune system both indirectly and directly, meaning fewer colds, etc. We know it increases self-esteem, and it's a natural antidepressant. It lowers blood pressure. It makes you look and feel younger.

It increases intimacy in relationships and builds trust, not only on a psychological basis but through the release of the connecting hormones mentioned above.

A word of advice: having a healthy sex life requires knowledge, so get some education. Without this, sex can cause anxiety and frustration, but learning to be open with your partner can build a stronger connection with them.

The message is simple. Having a sex life is healthy and beneficial. Don't stress if you don't have one, but if you do, take it seriously and work at keeping it strong and fulfilling. Age is no barrier!

Your To-Do List
- Understand that movement and exercise are not optional extras for health.

- Reintroduce movement into every daily activity that you are able to.

  - Approach exercise like you approach cleaning your teeth. Make it part of your morning habit.

  - You need to set aside fifteen minutes per day. That's it!

  - If you don't like exercise, keep it simple and keep it short.

- Take every and any opportunity to walk if you can. Yes, use the stairs.

  - The currently recommended minimum of 10,000 steps (about four miles) should actually be somewhere between 6,000 and 7,000 (about three miles). But the more steps the better.

- Forget the three-days-per-week deal. Just do it every day.

- Mix it up.

  - Yoga works and anyone can do it at home in fifteen minutes.

  - Choose sports that use every muscle. Swimming, tennis, badminton, and rowing machines are good examples.

  - Make sure you do some strengthening exercise: push-ups, sit-ups, and squats all use your body weight and gravity.

- Join a clan of people with a similar interest. Exercise is easier and more enjoyable in company.

- Remember exercise needs to be functional; it needs to enhance your life, so choose activities that promote strength, balance, and coordination in a way relevant to you. If you can get professional guidance, great. If funds are a challenge, consider a CrossFit group.

Make sure to add exercise as part of your daily routine. When you do, you will notice almost immediately how good you feel!

Your plan should now be taking more shape for the first two headings: Diet and Exercise. The next element sounds like it should be the easiest—after all, you just have to go to bed—but getting good sleep isn't always as easy as it sounds. Chapter 5 will tell you how you can improve sleep to feel better.

GET SOME SLEEP

· ·

Let's look at a few sobering thoughts that drive home the human cost of a lack of sleep:

- US kids get about two hours of sleep less per night than in 1920—and their physical and mental health, as well as grades, show it!

- In any given month, about fifty-six million US drivers admit to being drowsy when driving.

- One in five car crashes are due to this drowsiness.

- It's estimated that eight million people actually fall asleep when driving (micro-sleep) each month.

- That's a million crashes per year, with half a million injuries (55,000 of which are serious injuries with long-term effects), and about 7,000 deaths.

Sleep...Or Die

As you can see from the numbers, sleep is a matter of life or death. Dramatic statement? No, it's a fact!

Although a relatively new area of investigation, neuroscientists and researchers from many disciplines have discovered the enormous importance of sleep to your health. Psychoneuroimmunology, the study of how our mental state affects our immune and nervous systems, shows the role of sleep in restoring the neuro-immune system.

The preventative role of a regular, healthy sleep pattern on premature aging and disease is profound. Quality sleep is not an optional extra; it's a health and lifesaver.

If that is the case, why is an estimated 70 percent of the US population significantly sleep deprived? The answer is complex but is primarily due to the invention of electricity and the evolution of electronics.

Before we can talk about how to get more—and better—sleep, let's first look at why we sleep and the effects sleep (or the lack thereof) have on our bodies.

THE IMPORTANCE OF SLEEP

Why do we sleep? That's an excellent question, and the short answer is we don't know. All we can say is that pretty much every organism on the planet that scientists have studied undergo regular periods that can be recognized as "sleep." Our brain, with its central timekeeper, and every cell in our body follow a circadian rhythm—a twenty-four-hour waxing and waning of activity. Immune cells are no exception, and neither are the cells of our bacterial colonies. The importance of this is that there is an optimal time to do things like eat and sleep. Disrupting the rhythm with travel and night-shift work has profound effects on the body.

Clearly, sleep is essential. If you think about it, spending seven to eight hours asleep means that we spend approximately one third of our lives in a vulnerable state. You are unable to defend or protect yourself while sleeping. If we and other organisms place ourselves in this defenseless state, there must be a significant and crucial biological reason for us to do so.

· ·

To sleep, we need to be in a safe and secure place, both physically and emotionally.

· ·

We have discovered which parts of the brain are responsible for making us sleep and keeping us awake. Neuroscientists have clearer maps of the neural pathways and networks that link sleep to overall health, both physical and mental, as well as the role of sleep in memory and learning.

Once we wake and our brain kicks into daytime overdrive from nighttime restoration mode, we start to store by-products of the processes involved in energy production. Although the brain weighs about three pounds, representing only 2 percent of body weight, it uses 20 percent to 30 percent of the body's energy per day.

Adenosine, one of the chemicals produced as a by-product of energy production, begins to build up in the reticular activating system (RAS), the area in the brain that makes us alert and awake. As the levels of adenosine increase during the day, it reaches a critical point where the nerve cells in the RAS send signals out to the rest of the brain to slow down and go to sleep. Caffeine works by delaying this process. That's why many people who consume caffeine later in the day struggle to fall asleep.

This is particularly true in adolescent brains. Who consumes a lot of high-energy drinks with tons of caffeine? Teenagers! No wonder they are awake into the early hours of the morning.

During sleep, our brain literally washes itself down in the same way that city workers hose down the street and sidewalks during the night, clearing away the garbage and debris from the day before. This process removes the toxins that build up while the brain is busy when we are awake. It is crucial to brain health. Sleep appears to prevent the buildup over time of the specific chemicals and proteins that cause dementias, such as Alzheimer's disease. Put simply, lack of sleep is associated with premature aging of the brain and the risk of early dementia. These products also promote inflammation and changes in the behavior of the supporting glial cells, affecting mood and learning.

Sleep is crucial for memory and the formation of new concepts and problem solving. The idea that I can "sleep on it" and create new ideas or solve a challenging problem is correct. During sleep, your brain processes new information and integrates it with old knowledge, which changes your understanding of the world and modifies your constructs of how it works.

We need adequate sleep to be able to maintain concentration and focus. This is not confined to learning new things, as would be the case in school and college students, but is also essential to performing automatic tasks like driving. When we do not have enough sleep, we miss many visual clues that alert us to what's going on around us. This is one of the reasons the lack of sleep leads to increased accidents, especially in cars. Making matters worse, lack of adequate sleep slows your reaction time from a split second to actual seconds. This effect is true of everyone: pilots, athletes, air traffic controllers, along with many others.

Our ability to reason and problem-solve, along with the capacity to make rational decisions and apply sound judgment, is also severely decreased by lack of sleep. The issue with all these impairments is that even small amounts of sleep loss have a detrimental effect.

It is important to recognize that you will be totally unaware of this loss of efficiency, perhaps until it is too late. The brain is not equipped to monitor these changes brought about by nervous system fatigue! I suspect that evolution did not allow for this because for millennia, and until very recently, we all slept more than seven hours.

Our mood is also profoundly influenced by sleep. Less sleep means more emotional swings, meaning we become more erratic in how we feel. Poor sleep makes you much more prone to anger and irritation, as well as anxiety changes affecting all ages equally.

SLEEP AND YOUR BODY

We know that many processes occur throughout the body while we sleep, including functions that are involved in resetting many basic metabolic processes through the repair of cells and their chemistry.

The heart, which pumps the blood around your body, rests during sleep. Our pulse rate slows, and our blood pressure falls. Lack of sleep disrupts and can even prevent this necessary recovery period, increasing your risk of heart disease and high blood pressure. Sleep apnea is well recognized as being one of the leading causes of high blood pressure. It's reported that heart attack rates go up for a few days after the springtime change, as we lose an hour of sleep and adjust to the new time.

Lack of sleep is also known to increase your risk of obesity and diabetes. A lot of people think that sleep apnea is caused by being overweight. Actually, the opposite is true: sleeping poorly is one of the major causes of being overweight. The correct functioning of fat cells in our body is affected by disrupted sleep. Lack of sleep increases leptin production. It also makes the cells insulin resistant, leading to sugar intolerance, pre-diabetes, and diabetes itself. We know that even in fit, healthy, young people, two to three nights of badly disrupted sleep produce pre-diabetic pictures in blood chemistry!

We also know that lack of sleep has a significant negative influence on our immune system, increasing your risk of infection and cancer.

Sleep also has a powerful impact on the levels of background inflammation in the body. Lack of sleep increases inflammation, resulting in accelerated aging and early onset of degenerative disease.

Driving all of this is the discovery that every cell in the body has its own circadian rhythm—an individual sleep-wake cycle that is independent of the main clock in the brain. These cycles need to be in sync—brain and periphery. Disruption as occurs with night-shift work or transcontinental travel plays havoc, increasing risks of all diseases. Part of the horrible feeling of jet lag and increased risk of head colds with long distance east-west travel is due to this.

The Architecture of Sleep

Sleep is a complex activity. It's not a matter of just shutting your eyes and waking up a few hours later. It is a process, and during the night, different things occur at different phases.

The early hours involve "deeper" sleep, with bursts of what are called sleep spindles. This is when we transfer knowledge from short-term memory to long-term memory storage. For learning to be efficient, we need sleep before and after a learning experience. This is both true of factual information, such as study in school or college, and acquiring physical skills like learning a new sport or driving.

Later in the night, deep sleep is short, and we have rapid eye movement (REM) sleep. REM is when we have our most vivid dreams. This is when the brain sifts through the physical and emotional experiences of our lives and sorts them like a filing system.

Both non-rapid eye movement (NREM) and REM sleep are essential for memory and learning. This includes attaching new ideas to your current way of thinking. So if you want to change your lifestyle habits, you need to be sleeping normally to allow the brain to incorporate these new ideas into your current belief systems.

SLEEP AND MEMORY

Sleep is crucial for memory formation. Normal sleep architecture is required for the brain to store and sort the various experiences of the previous day.

We have different types of memory. Facts related to learning seem to be stored during deep, NREM sleep, when information is transferred from a part of the brain called the hippocampus to the long-term stores in the neocortex. Final storage requires REM sleep to consolidate them for future use.

New information that the brain considers to be background knowledge is stored during NREM sleep. This is the information that we use to form ideas that shape our opinions about things. These are experiences where we might not remember the details, but the knowledge changes long-term beliefs or behavior.

We also need normal sleep to learn and retain new motor skills. There is good evidence that the brain will replay the new circuits thousands of times at super-fast rates during sleep to construct new and unique neural pathways and network connections consolidating the behavior.

NREM sleep is needed to permanently establish both fine and gross motor tasks. So if you want to learn a new skill, take up a new hobby, and shorten the time required to learn, you need to have normal sleep the night after your training event. Interestingly, the converse is also true: learning a new motor task seems to improve the quality and structure of NREM sleep. So practicing your physical hobbies, sport, or activities like a new piece of music on your guitar improves the overall quality of your sleep. Being active, taking exercise, or learning just about anything improves sleep quality and, in turn, improves your overall well-being and health.

Bottom line: if you want to improve your memory and learning abilities, be it for factual information or motor skills, good quality sleep pre- and post-learning has a significant impact.

Relating memory to stress, we know that high cortisol levels seen during chronic stress impede the expected transfer of information during NREM sleep.

Cortisol is one of the main stress hormones. It, like several hormones, follows a circadian (twenty-four-hour) rhythm. Stress affects this rhythm, and the nighttime fall does not occur. When cortisol is high, the structure of your sleep is altered and the transfer of information between the hippocampus and the neocortex is disrupted. There is an associated change in the structure of dreams, and the effect is that stressed people find it difficult to learn complex, conceptual information and new tasks.

SLEEP AND EMOTIONS

Just as learning, memory, and recalling information all require adequate sleep, your emotional well-being is equally dependent on getting some sound shut-eye.

If you interact with people who are sleep deprived both acutely and chronically, you will be aware that they are emotionally labile—less able to control their feelings, be it anger or sadness. This is particularly noticeable in adolescents, who need eight to ten hours of sleep. The issue of increased use of social media and highly caffeinated drinks with shortened sleep times may well be linked to the current epidemic of teenage depression, anxiety, and suicide.

There is almost no psychiatric process that is not affected by sleep or disruption of normal sleep processes.

This applies to all of us. If you are not sleeping properly for seven to eight hours, you are much more prone to depression and anxiety. Insomnia has been shown to precede episodes of major depression, and there is a well-documented link with bipolar disorders.

When sleep deprived, you are much less able to cope with daily living stressors and much more prone to emotional outbursts. All this is because sleep deprivation somehow affects the functioning of the frontal cortex and the amygdala, the areas of the brain involved in regulating our emotions.

SLEEP AND INFLAMMATION

It should be of no surprise to you after reading this far that sleep quality has a profound impact on your immune system. You will recall that the nervous system and the immune system are not separate; they are intimately entwined. If you don't sleep, your nervous system is unbalanced, and so is your immune system.

If you are sleep deprived, then you have a weakened immune system. This translates into more infections, especially viral infections, including head colds. But it also weakens protection against cancer cells. Natural Killer cells (NK cells), one of our key defenses against cancer, are significantly less active in individuals who don't get sufficient sleep.

If you keep cheating yourself on a good night's rest, one of the consequences of the dysfunctional immune system is an elevation of background inflammation. Even after a single night of insufficient sleep, blood levels of inflammatory chemicals are higher. One night! But in long-term or chronic insomnia, this inflammation has a corrosive effect on our health.

Researchers looking at students clearly demonstrated that the stress and loss of sleep around exam times powerfully impacts their immune systems with significant increases in viral infections, like head colds and flus, along with cold sore breakouts on lips. Those who become unwell also tended toward more severe illnesses that took longer to resolve.

Stress also reduces our healthy response to vaccines, making them less effective. This immune-suppressive effect occurs in part because of direct actions of the stress hormones on immune cells, but there is also an effect through alterations of the nervous system. Failing to get sleep means that you are much less likely to make an adequate number of antibodies and immune T-cells that give you protection against the disease that they are supposed to prevent. Ensuring you have a good sleep before and after your annual flu shot, COVID-19 booster, or other vaccines makes a big difference and will increase your protection.

SLEEP AND EXERCISE

Split-second decision-making and super-fast reaction times with perfect coordination may not be of great concern to most of us, but to top athletes, it is crucial—the difference between winning and losing.

Whether you are an athlete or not, sleep affects your athletic performance significantly on several levels.

Less than seven to eight hours of sleep decreases the ability to learn and indeed perform fine and complex motor skills. There appears to be a lesser effect on gross motor skills, but reaction times are reduced.

Cognitive abilities are decreased. The power of the brain to make split-second decisions is markedly diminished. Problem-solving skills are also lowered. All of this translates into a decrease in performance in many sports.

There is also good evidence that when sleep deprived, your risk of injury increases. There are several causes, mostly related to those mentioned above. However, one is related to muscle function. Lack of sleep decreases muscles' ability to store glycogen (fuel), making them faster to fatigue and reducing muscle reaction time. So yes, you are correct if you have noticed that you have decreased athletic performance after a poor or short night's sleep.

If you are working on losing or maintaining reduced body fat and maintaining lean body mass, sleep deprivation leads to loss of muscle rather than fat. If you sleep less than seven to eight hours per night, 70 percent of your weight loss will come from muscle!

For men, reduced sleep also means reduced testosterone. If you are a regular five-to-six-hour per-night sleeper, your testosterone will be that of someone ten years older. Perhaps it's not an issue in your twenties and thirties, but it's a big deal at fifty and sixty. Not only will your physical strength and muscle mass diminish prematurely, but libido and sexual abilities decrease also.

. . . .

If you are working on your fitness or sporting performance and skills, setting the alarm for an early morning training session and cutting short your sleep is a bad plan. Same thing if you are trying to lose fat and be leaner. Insufficient sleep sacrifices muscle, not fat. Go to bed earlier and wake naturally. There will be significant physical gains.

. . . .

Now let's look at how much you need and some ways to improve your sleep.

How Much Sleep to Get and What Affects It

When you hear that you should get some sleep, you may think, "But I'm not tired!" Tiredness and sleepiness, however, are not the same things.

Tiredness means that you are feeling low energy or fatigued but do not need sleep. We can be tired for lots of reasons even if we have been getting sufficient sleep.

Sleepiness, on the other hand, is the feeling of needing to go to sleep. We all recognize this urge. Indeed, we often fall asleep. This is a primary drive that occurs when we are sleep deprived. Micro-sleeps, which happen when you are in this state, are the cause of many accidents. Scary but true, you may not even be aware that you fell asleep for a couple of seconds.

If you sleep for only four hours, your brain functions in the same way as someone who is approaching or just over the legal safe limit of blood alcohol. Your reaction times and problem-solving skills are thus the same as someone who is legally drunk. That's a sobering thought—and one with real relevance. One US study showed that allowing teenagers to get an extra hour of sleep, because of later school start times, reduced the fatality rate from car crashes by 75 percent.

So how much is enough sleep? The current consensus is as follows:

- For newborns: 14–17 hours

- For infants: 12–15 hours

- For toddlers: 11–14 hours

- For preschoolers: 10–13 hours

- For school-aged children: 9–11 hours

- For teenagers: 8–10 hours

- For young adults and adults: 7–9 hours

- For older adults: 7–8 hours

Surprised by those numbers? You shouldn't be—and you should strive to hit the low end of the range as your minimum goal.

But how can you hit the necessary amount of sleep for your health?

You have probably heard the words "sleep hygiene" and wondered what they mean. Well, the term encapsulates the key aspects of giving yourself a fighting chance of getting sufficient, quality sleep.

To be able to sleep, you first need to create a sleep opportunity, meaning seven to eight hours allocated to sleep. But in addition to the allocated time, you also need a place that is conducive to allowing you to nod off—and stay asleep, undisturbed.

To get good sleep, you require a safe, quiet, cool, and dark room. That means no TV or other distractions with light, other than your chosen podcasts or lecture (more on this in an upcoming section). Cool means sixty to sixty-seven degrees Fahrenheit. Quiet means put your snoring partner, if you have one, in another room, buy earplugs, or change them (the partner that is). Dark means thick curtains or equivalent. Safe is self-explanatory.

There is one thing you can do to make a significant change in your health with little to no effort: go to bed an hour earlier and get your average sleep times up to seven or eight hours. Sleep, that thing we do without being aware of, is not just something that is an inconvenient part of life. It is life! Not sleeping for seven hours a night has profound and life-altering effects. All are detrimental.

Sleep is the "lazy" person's way of improving their health. No aspect of your body function is untouched. Mental, physical, and immunological well-being are dependent upon sleep. Also included are your weight, your digestion, your capacity to learn, store memories, and information. Your mood and even your personality.

Let's look at what can affect those precious hours.

LIGHT

Probably the single most damaging change in modern life is the introduction of artificial light—specifically electric light in its many forms. Until the advent of fire, there was sunlight and nightlight—darkness. Our body and brain evolved around this single fact.

Melatonin, which is primarily produced in the pineal gland located in the center of our brain, controls sleep behavior throughout the body. It also has a profound effect on immune cell behavior. Melatonin production rises quickly with the setting of the sun and transition to night. This prepares the cells of the body to enter sleep preparation mode.

Unlike sunlight, and indeed oil, wax, and gas lamps, light derived from many electric bulbs and electronic devices have a great deal of blue spectrum light—a strong inhibitor of melatonin production. What this means is that, unlike our ancestors living over 150 years ago, we inhibit normal melatonin production right up to bedtime. Indeed we now continue this exposure in bed by reading on a tablet or other electronic device, or worse, watching TV shows or movies.

Not only does the amount of "cold" blue-dominant light matter, but the overall brightness matters as well. Think of how light naturally transitions outside your home at sunset. You need to replicate this in your home. Dim the lights a few hours before bed. Switch to warmer, softer, red-predominate light sources. You will be doing your bit to reduce electricity consumption as well—a feel-good-about-yourself bonus.

ALCOHOL AND SLEEP

If you drink, have you ever wondered why you seem to wake up earlier than usual after a fun night out? The answer is that sleep is an active process run by specific circuits in the brain. To have a restorative and health-enhancing sleep, all the correct programs need to run to completion, but alcohol is an anesthetic or brain depressant. In simple terms, it turns off the circuits that run your brain's sleep programs. *Alcohol is the poison of sleep.* Although there is individual variation, this effect occurs at surprisingly low levels of blood alcohol.

. . . .

To ensure good sleep, drink modestly and in the early evening.

. . . .

Here is how this works. Drinking alcohol raises the blood alcohol concentration. This level will continue to increase while you are drinking. At the same time, the liver is metabolizing the alcohol and turning it into fat. This process lowers the blood alcohol level. The average person can convert one unit of alcohol per hour.

One alcohol unit is 10 ml or 8 g of pure alcohol, which is equal to a one-ounce (25 ml) single measure of whisky (ABV 40 percent), or a third of a pint of beer (ABV 5–6 percent), or half a standard (175 ml) glass of red wine (ABV 12 percent).

So if you drink two glasses of wine (four units) over one hour at dinner at 7:00 p.m., you metabolize one unit during that time. At 8:00 p.m., you will still have three units left to break down. If you go to bed at 11:00 p.m., you will have a zero blood alcohol level. That's fine.

But let's say you have a cocktail (two units) at 6:30 p.m. Then three glasses of wine over dinner (six units) and an after-dinner drink (two units). All finished by 11:30 p.m., when you go to bed. That's ten units over five hours. During this time, you will have metabolized five units, leaving five units to go at bedtime. You will not have cleared it all until 4:30 in the morning!

You might ask why this is a problem. It is true that when you drink alcohol you will have a shortened sleep latency, meaning that you fall asleep faster. It's the reason so many people have a nightcap. You will also have a deeper sleep for the first few hours. But some of the vital restorative processes are switched off. Your NREM stages have abnormal structure.

Then there will be a rebound during the second half of the night. Your sleep is lighter than normal. You spend more time in abnormally light REM sleep. This means you may have micro-awakenings of which you are not aware. You may well wake up at 4:00 to 5:00 a.m. and be unable to go back to sleep.

So normal dream sleep, both REM and NREM, is disrupted. This matters because a lot of important things happen during dream sleep. One is the restoration of serotonin, the happiness neurotransmitter. If you do not restore normal levels, you often wake up feeling blue after a few drinks the night before.

But there are broader consequences. Even minimal amounts of alcohol affect the biological clock—the parts of the brain that control our circadian or twenty-four-hour biological rhythms. Every part of your body is affected by this: the neuro-immune system, numerous important hormones, our guts and liver, and even our mood and sex drive. Recall that this clock needs to be in sync with the micro-clocks in the 160 trillion cells in our body. Yes, those of you who are still awake will recognize that this number must include the bacteria in the microbiota. Indeed, they follow a circadian sleep-wake cycle just as we do.

Alcohol also affects our production of melatonin, which is crucial for normal sleep. Even modest amounts of alcohol before bed decreases production by up to 20 percent. That not only contributes to damaged sleep architecture but also suppression of your immune system.

Alcohol also affects the production of adenosine, increasing the speed of its production. Remember this chemical builds up slowly during the day and makes you sleepy in the evening. Alcohol increases adenosine production in the brain and is the reason why you feel sleepy in the afternoon after drinking at lunchtime and have a shorter sleep latency at night. It's also why many mixed drinks contain some caffeine to counteract this. Rum and Coke, or RedBull and vodka, for example.

So when is the best time to drink? Alcohol is cleared from the body most efficiently in the late afternoon and early evening. Think Happy Hour.

Last, on this topic, a hangover is a disease state. We all have heard the expression when walking into a party, "pick your poison." Literally, it's the truth. Besides everything discussed about alcohol so far, the products that alcohol is turned into and the congeners (other chemicals that make each drink what it is) are in general poisonous to the body at worst and metabolically disruptive at best. Overall, the clearer and cleaner the alcohol, the less likely the congeners will add to the poisoning.

I know this all sounds like a buzz killer, and perhaps it is, although it's not my intention to sound like a boring, anti-alcohol fanatic. But think about it: if you went to a restaurant and ate a meal with just water, then woke up in the morning feeling the way you do after a "great night out" with a few too many drinks, would you ever go back to that restaurant? No! Chances are you might complain, and almost certainly you would not recommend the place to your friends and family!

Yes, we all like a drink, and why not? I just ask a simple question: why do you drink? If the answer is a couple drinks to enjoy with friends, or because I like this particular wine, go for it. If it is ever because I need a drink, I'd recommend you think hard about your reasoning.

SLEEP MEDICATION

Taking sleep medication, although tempting and widely prescribed by a lot of doctors, is not really the answer.

Benzodiazepines, like Diazepam or Lorazepam, have a lot of problems associated with them. Other than short-term use for sleep in people who are acutely emotionally distressed from the loss of a loved one or a similar situation, they are to be avoided.

The "newer" meds, such as Zolpidem, do not produce normal sleep. You may feel like you slept, but measures of daytime psychometric tests do not show improvement, although some benefits have been shown in other areas of brain functioning.

. . . .

There is a solid and growing body of evidence that the best form of treatment for insomnia is cognitive behavioral therapy for insomnia (CBT-I). There are several online apps available that guide you through the CBT-I process.

. . . .

My own technique to return to sleep, which is now used by many of my patients, is to have a lecture or short podcast preloaded on YouTube or something similar. It must be interesting enough to catch your brain's attention, but not too interesting, and no more than twenty to thirty minutes long. Just listen to it and you will be surprised at how often you quickly fall back to sleep. I have listened to hundreds of hours of my Buddhist spiritual teacher in my sleep. His name remains a secret because he is not really that boring!

One of the issues regarding the management of sleep issues is that most doctors are poorly educated in this area. They really don't recognize that sleep disorders come in many different forms. The one-medication-fits-all solution is outdated and incorrect.

Your To-Do List

- You need seven to eight hours of quality sleep if you are an adult.

- Sleep hygiene is critical.

    - Make your bedroom a place for sleep, not an extension of your TV room.

    - Transition from day to night by starting to dim household lights two hours before bedtime.

    - Make your room dark. (If you use a night-light, remember to make it red, not blue.)

    - Electronic devices, including your tablet, Kindle, and phone, all produce blue light, which prevents melatonin, the sleep chemical, from being produced. Get rid of the gadgets, TV, and screens in the bedroom. TV in a bedroom is associated with a loss of around two hours of sleep per week.

- Read a book or listen to something before going to sleep. No screens.

- Enjoy a warm shower or bath before bed. A cooling body is a sleepy body.

- Create the correct temperature. Best is 60–67° F (15.5–19.5° C).

- Ditch your alarm! Set a bedtime and stick to it. Set it at a time that allows you to wake naturally without an alarm. Alarms start your day with a stress response.

- If you suffer from insomnia, the rule is no caffeine after lunchtime. This includes coffee, tea, hot chocolate, and caffeinated sodas, as this represents on average four to five hours of sleep loss per week.

- Alcohol is the poison of sleep, especially late in the evening. Drink small quantities at most two to three nights per week.

- If you have insomnia, try Cognitive Behavioral Therapy apps before medication.

- If you do wake up during the night, have a podcast, lecture, or book loaded onto your smartphone. (YouTube also works well.) When you wake, hit play, and listen—don't watch.

- Make sure you perform some physical activity during the day, practice a new skill, or gain some new knowledge.

- If you are trying to lose weight, then shortened sleep causes you to lose muscle, not fat.

One of the most helpful ways to get a better night's sleep is to manage stress. We'll discuss this in Chapter 7. But first, let's talk about another important element for better health: spending time with yourself, which I call Me-Time.

CHAPTER 6

IT'S ALL ABOUT ME-TIME

· ·

The saying goes, "If you fail to plan, plan to fail." As we saw in Chapter 1, if you want to change your life, you have to have a plan.

Part of my less-than-conventional career included a ten-year period when I flew commercially part time. I earned an Air Transport Pilot's license and a master's degree in aviation safety systems and human factors. My interest other than a passion for flying just about anything that flies, from canvas-covered biplanes to fast jets and gliders, was the psychology that leads to human error, and importantly from a practical standpoint, how systems, whether they're biological or organizational, interact.

When I would teach aircrew how to fly a mission successfully, it was always with the same format:

- Ask "What is the goal?"

- Develop a plan to achieve that goal.

When flying the mission, we kept asking an additional two questions:

- Are we on plan?

- Is the plan still relevant?

Take a minute now to evaluate your plan, and fill in anything that has changed as a result of your reading. You will notice that this requires headspace—something that comes when you have Me-Time.

What Is Me-Time?

For many, Me-Time is curling up in a chair with a good book and a cup of coffee, or retreating to a man cave, workshop, or garden shed. It's getting time alone to do something special and comforting to you. This is extremely good for you, but in my world, these activities do not belong in Me-Time; they belong in stress management (which we'll get to in the next chapter).

In the Five Elements, Me-Time is that part of your life that you set aside on a daily basis to check in with yourself. It is an active process. In its simplest form, it can be lying in bed first thing in the morning before the day invades your space and asking four simple questions:

- How do I feel physically?

- How do I feel emotionally?

- How do I feel mentally?

- Why do I feel this way?

. . . .

Me-Time is the process of taking stock of your life. It is an essential component of the Five Elements, and possibly the one you are least likely to practice.

. . . .

The purpose of Me-Time is to set aside some space every day to ask, basically, how am I doing, how am I feeling? Are the things I am doing helping me reach my goals? Am I on plan?

This book is in part a journey of change, and it should be clear to you by now that the best way to be successful is to have a plan.

One of the great challenges of our modern lives is that they are busy. We spend every minute of our day doing stuff. To my mind, one of the greatest losses over the last hundred years is the disappearance of reflective time.

In the world without modern electronic devices and light, there were significant periods of the day when people had to occupy themselves by *being* rather than *doing*. Artificial light is a very recent invention. If we go back 150 years, it was a luxury only enjoyed by the wealthy. The reality was that once the sun went down, most people went to bed and stayed there until it rose again at dawn. But we only need eight hours of sleep, so people had at least two to three hours during the night with nothing to do but live in their mind. Reflection time.

Electricity has transformed this. If we choose, we can live in full daylight twenty-four hours a day. We have extended our *doing* day to sixteen or more hours, and we have shut out our *being* time.

I'm going to suggest that you need to put it back. The health consequences are immense. One of the most immediate, which brings its own health benefits, is increased mindfulness.

Mindfulness

Me-Time helps develop the mindset of mindfulness. This means being aware of what is going on right now, inside you and all around you, being aware of your thoughts, feelings, and body sensations, and then linking them to the situation you find yourself in.

Mindfulness is learning to pay attention and take note of how we feel in various situations, such as after a good sleep, a certain meal, some exercise, or a period without exercise. This simple behavior leads us to change our lives, not because a doctor, pastor, or partner told us that something is "good" or "bad" for us. Instead, we want this mindfulness because we want to have that "feeling good" sensation. We can fail to recognize how we are getting on if we don't pay attention and ask ourselves how we feel.

A key component of mindfulness is that it is simply observational. It is without judgment. There are no *good* or *bad*, or even *right* or *wrong* thoughts or feelings, not even a sense of *helpful* or *unhelpful*. You practice mindfulness simply to be aware.

Why, you might ask, is this an element in this health program?

In 1979, Jon Kabat-Zinn launched a mindfulness-based, stress-reduction program at the University of Massachusetts medical school. Since then, several medical studies have demonstrated significant mental and physical benefits of mindfulness. It is now widely used across several branches of healing, including increasingly in mainstream medicine.

I've divided this activity into two types: passive and active mindfulness.

Passive mindfulness is learning to pay attention and take note of how you feel in various situations, such as after a good sleep, after a certain new activity, after some exercise, or a period without exercise, perhaps a change in diet. How you feel and react in different settings and situations, such as talking to a coworker, your boss, your partner, or friends. Being mindful helps you recognize and acknowledge the things that make you feel good and those that don't. As you practice being aware, paying attention if you wish, just like everything else, it becomes automatic. You build the mindfulness circuits. And as this happens, you will be surprised to discover how much of your life you had been sleepwalking through!

Active mindfulness, in contrast, involves a more directed process. It is primarily based upon meditation: a simple-to-learn technique that leads to changes in your brain that calm both the mind and body.

Mindfulness is simple to learn and practice. And it's free! Let's look at one technique to build mindfulness.

Focusing the Mind

Meditation and self-reflection are exercises of the mind that train it to be mindful. They are easy-to-learn techniques that lead to changes in our brain that not only teach our mind to watch us, but they also bring balance to the mind and body.

There are lots of names for this practice, but the more common are self-hypnosis in the west and meditation in the east. There are some definite differences, but the end point is really the same.

Both techniques are a focusing of the mind by using internal mechanisms. Basically, it's an induction of an altered state of mind. This focusing is like a telephoto lens zooming in on a part of a larger picture. Used properly, it allows us to observe and begin to understand some of the issues that shape our thoughts and attitudes and thus how we perceive and interact with the world.

Although the mind-state might be similar with hypnosis and meditation, the focus is slightly different. Hypnosis is truly focused on an event or a feeling. Meditation is a more generalized state of being aware of what is going on inside you. It trains the mind to pay attention to itself. Hypnosis is like surgery, where the cut is specific and the goal is defined. Meditation is more like a physician: the scope is broader and, in theory at least, should be more inclusive of the big picture.

· ·

The ability to meditate or self-hypnotize is quite different among individuals; about 50 percent find it difficult, while the other 50 percent finds it to be easy.

· ·

People who teach their mind to wander less, in particular those who teach themselves to stop ruminating or fretting, are healthier. They are less likely to get an infection and have longer survival times from significant diseases, including cancer.

We all know that if you go to the gym and lift weights, you will become physically stronger. If you practice basic meditation, the reward is not only a calmer mind and clarity of thought, but an increased level of awareness. Mindfulness is an increased personal awareness on a moment-to-moment basis without judgment.

Patients regularly tell me that they tried meditation but gave up because they couldn't get their mind to empty itself. Their head was still full of thoughts and worries. This is entirely normal. In meditation, we talk about the monkey mind: the idea that your head is going to be continuously filled with thoughts and ideas. What we are trying to do in meditation is create space so that we can train our mind to observe those thoughts and feelings without being hooked by them.

The goal is to train part of your mind to become an observer of the rest of you. This includes your thoughts, feelings, and bodily sensations. Why would we do this? Because most of us never sit quietly for long enough to be an observer.

Once you practice a little bit, you'll notice that you start to pay attention to what's going on with you throughout the day. This ability to become an observer-of-you while you are doing things allows you to change.

So how do you meditate? The simplest way is as follows:

Lesson One: Find a quiet spot. Sitting or lying down is fine. Just pay attention to your breath. As you breathe in, try to picture the word *in* in your mind; as you breathe out, just picture the word *out*. Try this for one or two minutes. That's it. Lesson one over. When your mind wanders, which it will, simply bring it back to the words *in* and *out*. The breaths will slow down and become longer as you practice.

Lesson Two: Start with lesson one, but this time we're going to extend our meditation to four minutes. After a minute of following your breath with *in* and *out*, you will find that all sorts of thoughts invade your thinking. That's fine. The goal this time is to try and let go of the thoughts rather than get hooked on them. That's it. Lesson two over. You are well on your way.

Lesson Three: Now that you can sit for four to five minutes, practice slowing your breathing down by counting slowly up to four, six, and eight during each inhale and exhale. Better still, add a short pause between the inhale and exhale and perhaps also between exhale and inhale. Take large full breaths, as deep as you can, and then exhale all the way out as far as you can go.

This very simple technique will bring balance to your autonomic nervous system and thus your whole body. It will literally calm you down. I know people think that it should be more complicated than this, but it is not. Just practice this for five minutes every day for a month. You will see for yourself!

Find a Community

Now it's time for something completely different. You might be surprised to hear me say that you should find a community in a chapter on Me-Time, but there it is.

This is one of those common-sense moments. We have evolved as group animals, and being healthy requires that we maintain these bonds. Our brains evolved to connect to other humans. Indeed our survival depended upon this fact. Living in isolation is a very recent phenomenon—less than 200 years old. Before that, most people never strayed far from their village. They lived in close-knit families and small communities, a system that had been in place for millennia. Travel was dangerous and rare.

Loneliness kills, and so cultivating membership in a group is critical. There are lots of tribes, and it does not matter which one you belong to—family, sports team, cooking club—but you need to be in at least one.

Related to that idea, vacations or holidays are good for your health. Surprised again? Taking a break can have measurable health benefits and has been shown to lower mortality rates. Time to just sit and relax is a big thing. It's a respite from the endless daily pressures of work, raising kids, and working on relationships.

It's also an opportunity to reconnect with yourself and with family or friends. One of the great truths in life is that people who have strong relationships with others are healthier. We need to be connected. Vacations allow us the space and time to do this.

Another way to connect is through cooking. Food and how we prepare it often defines different cultures and clans. We all recognize Italian or French cooking from Europe, or Thai, Chinese, and Indian cuisine from Asia. As culture plays an important role in health, cooking plays a role in psychological well-being.

On every continent, we celebrate special festival dates during the year. In the US, people look forward to Thanksgiving, and in Europe, there is the Christian celebration of Christmas; the Jewish community celebrates Hanukkah; the Chinese celebrate New Year, and in India, they celebrate Diwali. These celebrations share significant common themes. They bring people of the same culture together, most particularly families, and they all have traditional foods and dishes unique to that festival.

They also share something else: on the whole, happiness and laughter. Members of the family come together to prepare culturally traditional meals in styles unique to that family. These meals are typically produced in a cooperative and mutually supportive fashion, which is an important bonding process that not only builds relationships within the group but has profound impacts on individual members' well-being.

Even in our daily lives, we often meet for coffee, go out for a meal, and have business meetings over dinner. Special foods that are not part of our daily diet are a common theme to these events. (Most people don't propose over McDonalds!)

So the preparation and cooking of food serves a function over and above its nutritional value. It is an important component of defining a clan and its culture. As my grandmother used to say, "A little bit of what you fancy does you good." And what most of us fancy is our mother's traditional cooking.

Your To-Do List

- Take some Me-Time every day.

- Practice mindfulness.

- Learn to meditate.

- Make space to sit quietly and breathe each day for a few minutes to calm and collect yourself.

- Then actively practice full-breath breathing.

- When calm, spend a further five minutes getting in touch with yourself, checking in, and asking, "How do I feel physically, mentally, and emotionally, and why?"

- Join a like-minded family or clan to assist you with these behaviors.

Me-Time is powerful medicine, and by now you should not only be feeling better, but you should have a much better idea of how well your plan is working. There's still one more element to learn about, and it's the topic of Chapter 7: Stress Management.

CHAPTER 7

MANAGE THAT STRESS

· ·

There is a Chinese story that I like very much and frequently share with people:

A teacher is walking along a river path with his pupil. The pupil is unhappy and worries about lots of things. He recognizes that his worry is unhelpful. He asks his master what to do.

The teacher points at a small rock on the path and instructs the pupil to pick it up and hold it in his hand. They continue to walk.

After a mile or so, the rock, although small, is becoming uncomfortable to carry. Another mile after that, and the pupil's arm muscles are hurting. Eventually, the pupil says to his teacher, "The rock is heavy, and my arm is hurting."

The teacher turns to him and says, "Well, put it down."

We choose to carry so much of the past with us—past insults, failures, supposedly missed opportunities, and so on. They are like the rock: insignificant at the beginning, but the more we hold onto them, the more they bother us and weigh us down.

The solution is simple. Let them go. Put them down. Does holding onto these things make your life better, fuller, happier? No, clutching them and keeping them alive has quite the opposite effect. It leads to frustration, anger, and resentment. The end result of this is damage to your health.

Can you change the past? No. Will holding on to the insulting comment made by your Aunt Agnes at Christmas twenty years ago help you? No. Yes, your hurt and anger were justified then. But for twenty years? Nope. Hanging onto all this made it grow. Who is getting damaged? You.

Let it go!

Stress, the Silent Killer

It is a fact that stress kills.

Can you really die from a broken heart? Yes, you can, from Takotsubo cardiomyopathy, the broken heart syndrome. This condition is caused by severe emotional stress, such as breaking up with or losing a loved one, and can occur even in the healthy hearts of young people.

Does stress really cause you to die early or suffer from an increased burden of physical and mental health issues? Yes, it does.

Can childhood stress and adversity increase your risk of mental and physical illness later in life? Again, the answer is yes.

The common theme? Well, you know the answer now. You have learned the why. The mind and body are connected. Psychoneuroimmunology explains how thoughts and attitudes, along with the neurological, immune, and body-wide neuro-immune scars of our childhood and life story change the functioning of these critical housekeeping systems of the body. Let's fill in some further details.

Stress is part of life. There is no escaping it. In fact, stress in moderate amounts and if handled properly is actually good for you. It forces you to do something in an attempt to diminish it. Want to pass an important test? Stress will typically motivate you to study and achieve your goal. But—and it's a big but—how you handle stress, in particular chronic stress, is the difference between life and death, sickness and health.

Stress produces strain. It's not stress itself that kills you; it's the strain that it places on the body and mind. The good news is that you can engineer your life in such a way that you can protect yourself against the strain, just as engineers design a bridge to not only withstand the day-to-day wear and tear of normal traffic over many years but also regular storms and the occasional hurricane.

You can acquire simple skills and adopt some easy-to-learn habits that we know protect you against the physical, emotional, and mental damage of stress. The key ones are, of course, a healthy diet, regular exercise, adequate sleep, and self-reflection, prayer, or meditation. (Sound familiar?)

Questions concerning your perceived stress levels, along with inquiry into common stressors, need to be part of every medical doctor or healthcare provider's basic assessment when they meet you. As you will discover, there is a large and growing body of mainstream scientific evidence demonstrating that an individual's psychological makeup, which plays a significant role in how they handle the stress of life, has very real consequences for their general well-being, health, and lifespan.

· ·

Stress affects whether you become ill and what happens if you do. Stress affects how you heal from injury and operations. If your healthcare team does not ask you about stress in your former and current life, they are missing a vital part of your story.

· ·

The Stress Reaction

But what is stress anyway? And how does it actually affect our bodies?

Stress is anything that causes the body or mind to be pushed out of balance, out of their comfort zones. It can be in the form of emotional stress: loss of a loved one, break up of a relationship, bullying at work or school, being rejected by people around you, or by society in general because you are different.

It can be psychological stress: too many hours at work, not enough money to pay the bills, the pressure of meeting a deadline or passing an exam, or perhaps trying to solve a problem that you think you don't have the knowledge to fix. It can also be caused by the way you think about yourself and the world around you.

Stress can also be physical: an illness or infection, a broken bone or injury, too much exercise, a marathon, insufficient sleep, or a lack of quality sleep.

All stress causes activation of our fight-flight-fright reaction. This is a single solution to danger in our lives. Our neuro-immune and neuro-endocrine systems do not differentiate the cause, so physical, emotional, and psychological stress cause the same internal responses.

The stress response is normal in acute situations, but long-term activation can be immensely damaging to our health. This process is driven through two key systems in the body: the autonomic nervous system (in this case, the sympathetic branch) and the neuro-endocrine system, which operates through the hypothalamic-pituitary-adrenal axis (HPA-Axis). These two responses are connected and overlap, but they work quite differently. Both lead to profound changes in the neuro-immune system.

The acute stress reaction is the one intended to protect you from immediate harm. There are three common responses: fight, flight, or fright (freeze). It is entirely automatic and is driven by the sympathetic nervous system. It is the adrenalin reaction. You feel anxious, your pupils dilate, your heart rate goes up, your muscles tighten ready for action, and your gut shuts down. If this occurs while having a cup of tea with your friend, when there is no tiger about to eat you or someone trying to stab you, we call it a panic attack. It's the feeling you get when you have a "near miss" in a car or someone frightens you. This whole reaction is lightning quick and totally outside your control, at least in the initial stages. You have a feeling of impending doom, and you are driven to act instantly. The entire process should be short-lived and lasts for about twenty minutes, at which point your adrenalin runs out. You will notice that it is a whole-body response, including your mind.

Recent research has suggested that acute stress, producing large amounts of noradrenalin, can actually suppress immune cell function, hampering the body's ability to fight infection and cancer. The sickness behavior I mentioned previously, rest and withdrawal, may be the body's counter response, an attempt to enhance the immune reaction by dampening sympathetic activity. Certainly, medical teams should do their best to reduce acute stress as much as possible in sick patients.

The chronic stress reaction is a little different. This reaction is slower and comes next. It is both a neuro-immune and neuro-endocrine response, involving nerves, immune cells, and hormones, the most important hormone being cortisol.

I think it is true to say that we all recognize that stress is bad for us. What most people don't realize is how bad it is. Have no illusion: stress is a killer.

We know that your risk of developing cancer or having a heart attack is much increased after a period of acute stress. A recent divorce or separation, loss of a loved one, and losing your job are all associated with increased disease.

· ·

Think of the word disease itself: dis-ease, lack of ease.

· ·

Chronic stress is equally damaging. Just about every known disease, infectious and noninfectious, is more common in individuals who are chronically stressed. We also know that stress in your childhood, and even during your time in the womb, has a profound effect on the rest of your life, increasing your risk of developing ill health and an early death. This implies, and indeed is now corroborated, that what happens in childhood molds and hardwires your body's systems for life.

For a long time, we did not know why, but now we do.

It all comes back to the neuro-immune system, the neuro-endocrine system, and the process they control: chronic inflammation. We understand the mechanisms through which acute and chronic stress leads to increased inflammation, and as discussed elsewhere, we know that inflammation is the cause of both mental and physical disease, premature aging, and early death.

Chronic stress is associated with significant changes in the way our brains work. It affects memory and our ability to manipulate new ideas. In other words, it prevents us from learning. At a very fundamental level, stress is one of the significant barriers to change.

We also know that both acute and chronic stress are associated with a significantly increased risk of anxiety and depression.

STRESS AND PSYCHONEUROIMMUNOLOGY

In the 1960s, an American psychiatrist demonstrated that immune system dysfunction altered behavior and could be the cause of psychiatric disease. He was completely shunned by the scientific community and labeled a quack. Unfortunately, he was completely correct.

In the late 1970s, a psychologist and an immunologist working together showed that it was possible to condition and modify immune cell behavior in a form of Pavlovian conditioning using taste. This work was a repeat of Pavlov's own work nearly seventy years prior.

Since then, a lot of scientific studies have shown how an individual's environment, psychological processing, and their neuro-endocrine response to their surroundings have a profound effect on their immune function.

As mentioned previously, we know that students in the middle of exams are much more likely to have colds and flus compared to their friends who are not taking exams. We also know that the percentage of students developing antibodies to a vaccine goes down significantly if they are vaccinated during periods of high stress, compared to matched groups who are not under stress.

This diminished response has also been demonstrated in caretakers looking after a spouse or a partner with a significant long-term disability—a group of individuals who are well-recognized as having chronic high-stress levels. These caretakers are not only more susceptible to illness generally, but they also have significantly reduced responses to flu vaccines. Most importantly, psychological support and intervention to teach them how to cope with their stress and diminishing strain lead to a normal response to vaccines.

Your risk of getting cancer goes up significantly after an event like divorce, death of a loved one, or loss of employment. Most of us know someone who gets cold sores or fever blisters around their mouth, aptly named because they occur after head colds or periods of illness, along with periods of stress. It's the same with herpes zoster, a recurrence of the chickenpox virus in individuals who are ill, run down, or older. The "weakened" immune system allows the virus to reactivate, causing the painful rash we know as shingles.

As previously discussed, the nervous system, which controls how we think and feel and integrates the body's various functions, and the immune system, which is our housekeeping/maintenance department, operate as one. Any change in either part of this "single system" influences the way the other part operates.

Thus acute and chronic stress, both physical and psychological, have a profound effect on our immune systems. And the immune system has a profound effect on our nervous system, including how we think and feel. This is psychoneuroimmunology, and it is the center of who we are, how we live, how much disease and ill health we have, and ultimately when and how we die.

STRESS AND MEMORY

The hippocampus is crucial for the formation of memories by transferring what you learned today to long-term storage centers during sleep. The right hippocampus is for visual memories; the left for the things we read and hear. London cab drivers have a map of this complex city in their heads and have a larger than average posterior hippocampus.

The hippocampus also links memory to other sensations like smell. It is part of the limbic system. It's a very old, in evolutionary terms, part of the brain that we share with other mammals and indeed other animals. This is also the part of our brain that generates emotions.

Damage to this part of the brain significantly increases your risk for early decline in mental function—dementia. Chronic stress has been demonstrated to cause this area of the brain to shrink. Interestingly, exercise not only slows this damage, but it can actually reverse it.

The stress hormone, cortisol, is anti-inflammatory. Thus, having high levels due to stress should protect the brain from inflammatory damage caused by stressors. Well, it turns out that excess cortisol produced by chronic stress has exactly the opposite effect in the hippocampus. It drives brain inflammation in this area and increases the damage. Cortisol literally destroys the part of the brain associated with memory formation and learning, and their connections to emotions. If you want to experience early dementia and shorten your life and healthspan, choose chronic stress as a lifestyle.

> Good news: Get rid of the stress and your hippocampus will stop shrinking. Exercise regularly and it appears to recover.

STRESS AND CANCER

Cancer is stressful. Very stressful. The impact of cancer is complex and affects every part of a patient's life. How a patient handles that stress and strain has very significant consequences. For those who find ways to manage stress, there appears to be an opportunity to live a better life and even survive longer than those who are not taught what to do.

My record survivor was a friend who had stage four (metastatic) bowel cancer. He should have survived only a couple of years, but he surpassed eleven years. He had modern medical therapy, and of course it played a very important role. But what made him so memorable was that we devised an aggressive plan to manage his reaction to his stress.

This plan included a significant element of actively managing his emotions and mood. It was challenging for him at times, but it worked. One goal was to hang on to his humor. He allowed himself to express his feelings, including frustrations, fear, and anger. He kept hope. He stayed at work. He wrote an excellent book, which was itself a powerful tool in his illness management plan.

Studies have shown that you can predict survival in cancer patients from several psychoneuroimmunological markers. When we cannot cope with a stress, we lose the normal, daily, rhythmic high and low levels of cortisol—one of the body's neuro-endocrine reactions to this state of being. Losing the normal rise and fall appears to predict shortened survival times.

If we look at sleep patterns, another marker of neuro-immune well-being, we find a similar pattern. Individuals who sleep poorly appear to die earlier than those who are able to sleep soundly.

Depression itself may not confer a higher risk of getting cancer, but it is a significant predictor of survival. Contrary to most people's beliefs, depression is not always a consequence of a terminal diagnosis. Sadness is normal; depression is not and should be aggressively addressed. Depression leads to negative thoughts framing the patient's reality by painting a defeatist picture of the world. It is in part related to altered responses of the immune arm of the neuro-immune system. Thus, it can be challenging to manage as cancer alters this system. This is another example of the importance of treating whole patients and not just their disease.

. . . .

Psychological intervention should be a critical part of any cancer patient's management plan provided by health and sickness care services. When was the last time your doctor asked you how you are feeling emotionally and mentally?

. . . .

STRESS AND TELOMERES

Chronic stress also damages another part of the most fundamental component of life: the DNA within our cells.

Telomeres are the covers on the ends of your DNA. Like the plastic ends on a shoelace, they protect the fragile strands of DNA from fraying.

In simple terms, measuring telomere length tells us how much your body has aged. When telomeres get to a certain length, they stop a cell from being able to renew itself. That's a problem because we need them to divide. That's how we repair our bodies during life. Once cells cannot replicate, we begin to die.

Senescent (non-dividing) cells also cause chronic inflammation by secreting inflammatory chemicals (cytokines). More senescent cells means more inflammation with a higher risk of losing your health and decreasing your lifespan.

Specifically, stress damages the ends of our genetic strands, shortening these telomeres. Chronic stress can add decades to your biological age, shortening both your healthspan and your lifespan. Telomere length is also affected by mood, chronic anxiety, and depression.

Stress from any source causes premature shortening by increasing something called oxidative stress in our cells, along with other damaging chemical processes. Physical, emotional, and psychological stress all have this effect, with a lot of variation among individuals.

There is, however, an important caveat: psychologists have noticed that the amount of shortening appears to be related to how an individual perceives stress in life rather than how much pressure they actually have in their lives. We are back to the concern of strain rather than stress itself causing the damage.

Strain is something that can change. Mindfulness makes us aware of our reactions and then offers an opportunity to alter how we think and behave. Living a healthy lifestyle, such as suggested in this book, helps us manage and protect ourselves against the strain placed on the body by stress.

What Causes Stress?

Research in psychoneuroimmunology is beginning to unravel the biology of how our childhood, and indeed childhood trauma in all its various types, leads to increased risk of many diseases in adult life.

Consider the modern human experience from the moment of birth and the first few weeks and months of life—and then compare it with images from nature.

Have you ever seen a film of an ape taking its newly born offspring and placing it into a plastic crib? No, of course not. The moment that the infant is born, it is physically nurtured by the mother holding it close to her chest. This is not just a matter of feeding; it is a skin-to-skin process of bonding and caregiving. I mentioned the importance of this before in the section on exercise.

That's what you see on the outside.

In the brain, there is a whole neurobiological process of new circuits and wiring being laid down. It is the beginning of the development of a healthy ape. Note that it is a physical event; being held is the driver of the development of these circuits and networks. It is touch, smell, and hearing that make this process happen. The infant learns to read the mother. For the first few days, and even weeks, the baby ape never leaves the mother's physical presence. It eats and sleeps right there on her chest or somewhere on her body.

Now consider the modern human experience. Picture a hospital, the image of a crib or cot, and think about the separation of newborn from mother so they can rest.

We get it wrong from the moment we are born.

Almost all psychological and psychiatric conditions are much more common in adults who had challenging childhoods. Generally, the worse the stress, the higher the risk. Drug addiction, alcoholism, depression, and in particular chronic anxiety are all much more common in those who experienced difficult childhoods.

This is also true of the so-called functional illnesses—(IBS), fibromyalgia, palpitations, and other chronic, somatic pain syndromes.

Childhood adversity can have a profound psychological impact in the form of disordered thoughts and feelings about not only ourselves but the world around us. Even relatively short-lived traumatic events can have significant effects on a person's future health.

Perhaps that makes instinctive sense, but what if I told you that diabetes, high blood pressure, obesity, cancer, heart disease, and many neurological conditions and diseases of the intestine are all much more likely to occur in these individuals? In other words, the quality of your childhood and parenting predicts health and sickness levels for the rest of your life.

And it's not just your childhood. The ways in which you emotionally and intellectually navigate the challenges of your daily life play a major role in predicting how ill or healthy you will be. How you view the world and what type of conversation you have in your head has an immediate and direct effect on your physical health, both in the short and long term.

The key concepts to grasp here are that your childhood experience from the moment you are born influences the way the brain is wired and the way your immune system develops. If you grow up in a nurturing environment, your brain develops and is hardwired very differently than someone who experienced non-nurturing, abusive, or neglectful environments. In these situations, the brain spends a great deal of time in survival mode. It builds survival circuits, and these can be immensely problematic further down the line.

Of course, the reality is that very few of us grow up in a perfect nurturing environment, in part because of the structure of modern society. We have chosen a model where not only have we torn apart the structure of the village or clan, but we have destroyed the idea of family. We are no longer raised by a village but rather isolated units of two—and increasingly one—individuals who are often absent at work, and when physically present are too exhausted to be truly available to nurture children.

The fact is that many if not most of us suffer from some degree of childhood "trauma." The concerning issue here is that because of cultural drift, this is now accepted as the new norm. Thus, society struggles to recognize how far we have drifted away from the biological and psychosocial needs of a naturally developing human. Sadly, a great deal of damage was done by some strange theories promoted by early developmental psychologists whose ideas were based to some extent on the idea that humans are not really mammals. We are supposedly biologically different because we are the "chosen ones."

EPIGENETICS

Psychoneuroimmunology is beginning to deliver scientific understanding of how the events of your childhood leave scars in the neuro-immune system. This process is in part mediated by what is referred to as epigenetic changes.

The genetic code, which is hidden in the strands of DNA in each of our cells, is a shop manual that guides the manufacture of proteins in the body. These proteins are what we are made of. They drive the machinery of life. Our DNA strands contain the directions of how to build these structures.

Epigenetics is the process by which our environment and life experiences influence the way in which these instructions are read.

If you have an instruction manual, you have to open the page and read the directions. Our DNA code is 24,000 pages, each containing a set of instructions for a specific protein. If two pages are stuck together, you will never be able to open these pages and build that protein.

Simply put, epigenetics is the study of how the pages get stuck together. One of the causes is childhood experiences, while others are related to the way we choose to live our lives, whether we exercise, sleep well, and of course the type of food we eat. Stress has a profound effect on genetic code expression. These changes to the way the DNA code is read are sometimes permanent. The page will never become unstuck, and the effect is a lifelong change in some part of the functioning of the body.

. . . .

Several of these epigenetic changes occur in key parts of the brain that control the function of various body parts. They can change the way the body senses pain. They are in part responsible for several neuro-immune conditions, such as fibromyalgia, palpitations, and Irritable Bowel Syndrome.

. . . .

Childhood adversity may well produce epigenetic changes that increase your risk of cancer, infectious diseases, and noninfectious diseases like diabetes and high blood pressure.

Having an adverse childhood has a profound effect on your adult health and well-being, both physically and mentally.

Outsmarting Stress

Removing as much stress or strain as possible is key to allowing your thinking and attitudes to change. This is obviously relevant to how you construct your plan, so in the quest for improved health and well-being, managing stress is a crucial element.

To summarize what we have learned thus far:

Not all stress is a killer, but chronic stress can lead to strain, and this in turn damages your body and your brain.

Strain ages you prematurely because it damages your cells directly, changes your brain structure, and has a significant impact on your neuro-immune system. Anything that impacts your immune system and increases levels of background chronic inflammation is bad news. Chronic strain causes loss of the normal cortisol rhythms, leading to secondary metabolic issues, including weight gain and unhealthy fat distribution, muscle loss, and an altered microbiota and sleep patterns. This in turn leads to further derangement, and the fire is fed.

This process can be acute but is typically chronic. The problem with chronic stress is that the changes are slow and unfelt. Like a tap dripping into a bathtub, it will eventually fill the tub. As the change is slow, it goes unnoticed, and we accept each new phase as the new norm. Then, one day you wake up and the damage is done.

The solution is surprisingly easy. There are several spots where you can intervene. Of course, we all know that some things cannot be avoided, but you can at least identify and manage the stresses in your life.

First is to avoid the stressors completely. If you are in a bad job, look for a better one; a bad relationship, work toward fixing it or leave. If you find you constantly worry about something you feel you have to do in your life, ask yourself if you really need to do it. If it's not critical, then forget it. If you brood over old hurts and difficult events in your life, put them down and let them go.

The second approach is based in the idea that we frame our reality because of the way we view life. Understand that what you think influences what you feel and how you behave. Equally, how you behave will influence how you feel and think. These are all completely changeable and totally within your control. Indeed the only thing you *can* control are your thoughts and actions. The rest of life is outside of your control. Trying to manage and influence how the world around you operates and unfolds is an exercise in futility and a significant source of most people's stress.

The third is to understand the importance of play. It never occurred to me that there would be a play circuit hardwired into our brain, but one day I was listening to Jordan Peterson's lecture on the *12 Rules for Life*, and besides talking about lobster hierarchies, which are interesting in their own right, he mentioned play. It turns out that a super smart neuroscientist had discovered a play circuit in mammal brains. This is fascinating to me. Never mind the fact that rats have a giggle response if you tickle them; all mammals play. It turns out that play is crucial not only to normal neurological development, but that it may have a significant effect on your immune system as well by altering stress responses.

> While writing this book, I was standing in the kitchen early one morning and across the valley was a group of young lambs probably four to six weeks old. They had broken away from their mothers and formed a gang. For half an hour, I watched them racing each other up and down an old Devon bank. The fun thing was spotting the different characters. It left me with a warm and fuzzy feeling, and I headed out to work in an exceptionally good mood. Reflecting on this, I realized that it's pretty much always the case if you watch children or animals at play. There always seems to be an uplifting of mood and spirit. Those of us who live around animals will know they play, and they don't give up as adults.

We know that healthy play stimulates a child's mind and is crucial to not only social development but improves intellectual functioning and indeed an individual's IQ. As adults, we also need to remember how to play. Being playful improves our health through a variety of mechanisms, including the release of endorphins and other hormones that make us feel good. It strengthens relationships and bonds. It typically involves laughter and often physical exercise. We know it lifts mood and lightens us up.

Learning to be playful and seeking out playful and fun people is a critical part of stress management and has no downsides. Have fun!

And of course eat healthy, take some exercise, get your sleep, and enjoy some Me-Time—and manage your expectations.

EXPECTATION VERSUS ASPIRATIONS

What is the difference between expectations and aspirations?

If you think about it, when you become frustrated and even angry with life, a situation, or someone, it's likely because you had an expectation that was not met. The trouble with expectations is that there is a sense of entitlement. For example, if you go to the gym every day, then you expect to end up being much stronger. In reality, it may be that your body type isn't going to get you there. Then you become frustrated, and this frustration leads to stress—all because you had an expectation that was perhaps unrealistic.

I suggest that perhaps a better way to live is by having *aspirations*. This is a little different because there is a lack of entitlement. Aspirations come more along the lines of "I hope this is going to happen" rather than "I deserve for this to happen."

In truth, life almost never goes the way we expect, and so we have the potential to live a life filled with frustration because our expectations are not met. Furthermore, the degree of frustration that we feel is proportional to the distance between our aspiration or expectation and the reality of our life.

If you reflect on it just for a short while, the truth of our lives is that many and possibly most of our expectations and aspirations are not met. And even if they are, it is often not exactly as we had anticipated. My guess is it's another case of the Pareto principle or 80:20 rule. About 80 percent of the time, life goes its own way. The other 20 percent of the time, it might approximate our aspirations.

I'm not suggesting that if you replace the word expectation with aspiration that life is just going to go smoothly. But what I've noticed, as have others that I've worked with, is that living with aspirations takes the sting out of the issue when what we hoped for does not happen. We can significantly lower our level of frustration and stress if we can develop a "there we go again" attitude toward life.

Now, critics have said to me, "If you don't have any expectations, why would you get up in the morning?"

The answer is that an aspiration is still a goal. It's still something to get up for; it just implicitly suggests that we may not get there. This is no bad thing in itself because, in reality, life is mostly the journey and of course not the destination. Sadly, many of us forget this fundamental truth. As it is a truth, we might at least try and enjoy that journey.

This is part of being mindful: living now in the present without judgment, striving to accept the ups and downs of the day as they occur. Remember what goes up is coming down, and in reality, nothing is forever.

Your To-Do List

- Understand that life is stressful, and there's no escaping this! Accept this fact and actively protect yourself.

- Understand that stressors come in many forms: physical, emotional, and psychological. Recognize that your emotional and mental health are critical to good health, so take it seriously.

- Understand that drama is created by us, not by life. Work toward getting rid of the drama in your thinking. Try to stop catastrophizing.

- Change expectations (entitled) for aspirations (hope).

- Make your aspirations realistic to your actual life circumstance.

- Frustration and stress levels are proportional to the distance you place between your aspirations and the reality of your current situation.

- Stress is deadly, so you need a plan to deal with it. There are proven techniques to do so.

  - Learn to breathe. Sound silly? Well, it's not. One part of the stress reaction, acute or chronic, is shallow breathing. Slow, full breaths rearm the relaxation circuits in the body.

  - End the day with a set of positive thoughts. Something went right at some point today, however small.

  - Learn to laugh at life but most importantly at yourself. Humor and laughter change your response to stress. Don't take life too seriously. Nobody gets out alive anyway.

  - It really is true we can learn from rough times. Find the silver lining. Turn negative events into positive ones.

- Create a list of all your old grudges and hurts. Then put them down. They are old and done. They cannot be undone, so let them go. They are killing you, no one else.

- We create our own reality. Your thought beliefs and behaviors shape your world. Do yours increase your stress? Probably. So change them.

We've now covered all five of the essential elements for better health. Feeling better?

You should have a fully formed plan for each of these Five Elements, with concrete steps in place for reaching your goals. In Part III, we're going to begin to enact this plan in your life.

PART III

EXECUTING ON YOUR PLAN

. . . .

CHAPTER 8

BARRIERS TO CHANGE

· ·

Whenever we ask someone, including ourselves, to change, there is one common refrain: "I can't do it!"

Sound familiar? The words may be different, but the meaning is the same:

"I want to be slimmer, but I cannot eat differently."
"I want to be fitter, but I cannot exercise or find time to exercise."
"I want to sleep, but I cannot live without a TV in my bedroom."
"I want more Me-Time, but I cannot make time."
"I want to be less stressed, but I cannot change my life."

The truth is, we should replace "I cannot" with "I don't want to"!

When I suggest this to patients, after the initial flash of irritation of being judged, most will then smile and admit that this is probably true. They cannot change because they don't really want to change. After all, they are managing okay at the moment (sort of?), or indeed get pleasure (but not happiness) from their behavior.

And that's the point: getting by at the moment is easier than making substantial alterations to the way you live your life. The pursuit of pleasure often trumps the pursuit of happiness. (And, yes, there is a difference, as you will soon discover.)

But most of us need to change things in our lives. We know it and at some point come to the realization that we need to try. In truth, most of us even know what it is that we must do, and yet we can't get past the "I can't" conversation in our head. Let's look at why this happens.

Why We Struggle to Change

You might know or have already heard most of what I have written about in previous chapters, but you've never been able to implement those changes.

Most of us want to change something in our lives, but it's not that easy. We wake up one day and realize that we have wandered down a particular road. We recognize that it's not where we want to be. But heading in a different direction is very challenging. So what are the barriers to change, and how do we take them down?

The most significant are habits, bias, and fear of judgment. Let's take a closer look at each of these barriers to change.

HABITS

Familiarity feels good. It feels right. It's you.

Habits are hardwired into the brain.

As the brain develops, it learns, forming engrained circuits just like the wiring in your home. If you keep repeating something, these circuits become stronger. After a while, they become the preferred circuit, and a habit is formed.

Lots of habits are created incidentally without thought. Others are consciously programmed by our choosing repetition. What is essential to recognize is that the brain likes patterns of behavior. It's an efficient method of operating, and so once you build a strong circuit, it becomes the default and an automatic thought or action.

Most of what we do is habitual and subconscious, especially the way we react to just about everything in our lives. Speech and language, along with thought patterns and beliefs, walking, and playing a sport are all examples of persistent circuits. But so is the flash of anger and reflexive laughter, along with anxiety to certain situations.

Habits matter because they are barriers to making adjustments to your life. You feel uncomfortable when you break one. However, they can also be the key to change. You can develop new habits if you choose to. Central to being a "better" you is making this choice because you have to develop a deep desire to do things differently to be successful. Just as learning a language is challenging, so is learning a new skill or behavior. But persistence and practice will get you there. You took years to get here, so it'll take time and some perseverance to get onto and remain on your new track.

Imagine that your granny lives in the country. She's been in the same house forever. She likes gardening. For years, she has been pushing her wheelbarrow of weeds and grass clippings down the same path to the compost heap. The route is hard-packed earth and smooth with no stones. It's easy to push the wheelbarrow down this path.

Now we ask her to make a new path. It starts out difficult. It's bumpy and rough. Little rocks and grass make it hard work. But little by little it gets easier. Eventually we have a new path! Now she has a choice. The old path is so well used it will never fade completely; the new path is fine but if she stops using it, then it will overgrow pretty quickly, and she will find it challenging to use again.

Such are habits. Old ones die hard and frankly never really completely disappear. New ones need a bit of perseverance.

Can we change? Of course we can! We can all learn new skills, sports, or languages. We learn all sorts of things all the time—new facts, new information. What we are talking about here is learning new attitudes and behaviors. That requires an open mind, a degree of playfulness, and commitment to get over the initial hump.

BIAS

Bias—the subconscious way that our brain is wired to produce our view of the world—is also crucial to understanding why we struggle to change.

The reality of our lives is that we create stories and a mental model of the world around us. I'm not talking about holograms or other esoteric theories of the universe, just plain neuroscience. The way that we perceive and understand our interaction with the world is unique to us. It's shaped by genetics and epigenetics, our childhood experiences, and our subsequent life stories.

As we grow up, our brain develops hardwired circuits based upon experience and the environment in which it develops. After that, our view of life is reinforced by what happens to us. We pay more attention to things and events that our mind has decided are important to it. Often negative things, as these are greater threats to us. Thus we all have a natural tendency to see the negative side of life. It's a protective mechanism.

Bias is a bit like what happens with Google: the more you search certain topics, the more Google will provide information on this very same topic. The trouble with this is that it is not balanced, so you get to see less and less alternate points of view. This is why liberals cannot understand conservative perspectives and vice versa. Difficult to understand, but it's a psychological fact. We become programmed and locked into our own personal and unique reality. That's why even the most educated and intelligent individuals struggle to hear or understand alternative points of view.

This is bias. From the perspective of neuroscientists and psychologists, there are lots of specific biases. There's no need to get into the details here. All you need to know is that they exist, and this has very real consequences in relation to you changing your behavior.

The thalamus is the part of the brain that sorts incoming information and directs it to the correct area for processing. Various parts of the brain send information back to the thalamus, instructing it what to let through. In practical terms, this explains why we like certain types of faces or music. Our brains develop selective vision and hearing pleasing to it. But it's more than just physical events that are filtered. If we have a tendency toward being sad, our thalamus lets in information that supports the idea that the world is sad; equally, those with a happy disposition block these events and let in positive data.

If a baby is born into a family, suddenly there seem to be babies everywhere. Buy a new car or coat, and suddenly everyone seems to have the same car or coat. Of course they were always there, but our brain—happy with the new addition—suddenly selects these objects to watch. This is true in regards to all our interactions with the world. The fact is that our brain creates our own reality: our own bubble or silo.

This phenomenon applies to emotions and memories also. Our memories and how we store information are altered by our emotional state at the time of the event. Later, how we recall what happened can be altered by our emotions at the time of recall.

Thus we all experience a specific event in very different ways from other people who were present at the same time. This psychological phenomenon leads to family disagreements, fall-outs between friends and colleagues, along with incorrect imprisonments.

So as we grow up, we develop a unique picture of the world around us, and then the brain actively collects information to support this view. All this is being done unconsciously. The reality is that a lot of decisions that you make and actions that you take are carried out based on this very personal, biased, unconscious model of the world. It's pretty obvious that this has massive implications if you want to change because you are going to have to rewire some of these circuits.

By now hopefully you understand that the way you do this is by actually *doing something different*. Change comes through action, not thought. Thinking about things is the process that makes you want to change, but doing it is what changes you. It's crucial you understand this. No amount of visualization is going to get you to your goal. You can no more change your preference for certain foods by thinking about it than you can learn to drive a car by reading a book.

Changing attitudes about how you live your life requires learning new attitudes and habits and letting go of old ones. You are going to have to rewire your subconscious mind by actively acting out your new ideas and life choices.

> A quick reminder here: adequate exercise and sleep are critical to the process of changing your perception of the world and ultimately your core beliefs and opinions about things. Learning new skills and consolidating them through memory requires sleep.

FITTING IN

Around 70,000 years ago, a volcano erupted in what is now Indonesia. The fallout of this event reached all the way to Africa and Europe. It was an apocalyptic event that left large parts of the world covered in half a foot or more of ash and silica. As it occurred at the end of the last Great Ice Age, it appears to have prolonged this event. The world where humans were evolving became a more hostile environment with significant changes.

This appears to have contributed to a fundamental alteration in *Homo sapiens'* behavior.

There is evidence that supports the idea that this event precipitated an important evolutionary change in social interaction, the restructuring of human behavior from that of troops to that of tribes. Chimpanzees operate as troops. They are isolated from other groups, demonstrate territorial behavior, and generally interact with other troops of chimps aggressively.

Several diverse lines of research would suggest that following this mega-volcanic eruption—an event leading to significant climate change—*Homo sapiens* developed several traits that allowed us to survive, mainly cooperative behaviors. In other words, troops of early humans began to exchange things with each other. It is proposed that there were interactions within groups and between groups that were less aggressive and mutually helpful. The emergence of this type of cooperative practice allowed for survival in difficult times.

This move toward tribal or clannish traits, where individual groups saw themselves as related to other and indeed larger groups with an understanding that they have common goals, was a significant step forward for the human race. Beneficial, cooperative interactions among organisms within any ecosystem drive evolutionary change that supports survival of the entire system. This alteration in the way early humans interacted is perhaps what gave us the edge over our competitors for the ecological space we occupy.

We all recognize that within tribes there is a general consensus about unifying features. Think about Native American powwows. Individual family groups, which can be quite large, come together to exchange news and ideas and celebrate their common values and spiritual beliefs. Each family will have its own unique characteristics and idiosyncrasies, but they share sufficient common core values with the other family groups to make them a tribe.

Certainly, there is bickering and discord within a tribe, but typically serious conflicts are confined to those between tribes who are differentiated by different beliefs, cultural norms, and customs based in part on environmental influences.

What's this got to do with change? Well, several things.

The first is that our need to belong to a tribe goes back at least 60,000 to 70,000 years, a relatively long time in social evolution. As it occurred early in our modern human history, it runs deep in our psychological makeup and is hardwired in our brain. The basic neurological circuits were already present, laid down much earlier in the evolution of the mammalian brain and expressed as troop actions. But the subtle modifications leading to cooperation among troops, turning them into tribes, was the critical evolutionary step.

The way you live is dictated to a great extent by the rules and social norms of your tribe. As you will see in the next section on fear, what creates significant barriers to change is a sensible and realistic unconscious fear. If we change our personal behavior and break from the norms of the tribe, we will be ostracized. This is not just true of humans, but it's a very key component to the survival of animals in many mammalian groups. As individuals, we are fairly weak and vulnerable, but we have survived and been successful because we are tribal, and we work in cooperative groups. Being ostracized in evolutionary terms equals death.

It's very difficult to maintain a change or changes in your life that are significantly different from the group of individuals around you— your tribe—because your new behavior means you run the risk of no longer being a member of that tribe. If you live in a world of smokers, being a nonsmoker makes you an outsider; conversely, if you live in a world of nonsmokers, being a smoker makes you the one to be rejected. This is why society and culture play such an important role in deciding the health of an individual.

It is a significant barrier to change and leaves you with two choices: you either join a new group or try to influence and change the attitudes of those around you. These two options are not mutually exclusive. However, the initial way forward is indeed to join a new group.

One of the great benefits of social media is its ability to allow us to join with others who have similar ideas without having to physically leave our own group. We can find all the support we need online. We can interact, exchange ideas, and provide mutual support.

So as you begin to transform your life, one of the first things you need to do is to identify individuals who share similar goals. Then join that group. This is a doing thing.

As you find support from your new associates, it will become much easier to be a little different from those immediately around you, your family, and close friends. From a position of relative strength, you'll be empowered to try and change the attitude of others close to you.

And the best way to do this? Actions speak louder than words. Make your changes and let the results speak for themselves. Members of your immediate tribe may or may not join you in your choices. That's okay. Enjoy the support of those who share your goals—the members of your new tribe. As your life improves, those around you might see the reasons for this change and be tempted to join you!

FEAR

Another significant barrier to change is fear.

Fear is challenging. It's a very primordial feeling. It evolved to keep us safe and to prevent us from putting ourselves in danger.

One key fear is that of isolation or rejection. As discussed, our brains understand from a very early age that we are reliant on others. We need to belong to survive. We have our tribe, primarily family and friends, but we also have secondary tribes: football teams, clubs, and so forth. We're members because we conform to the general, defined rules. Instinctively, we know that if we change our lifestyle, we're out.

The possibility of rejection by the clan raises another, closely related fear: that of judgment. None of us like to be judged. It's a very unpleasant feeling. We don't like it when others judge us. We don't enjoy being judged by ourselves. (We'll examine this more in the next section.)

The third fear is the fear of change. We just don't like change. Don't worry about the psychology behind this; it's complex. Just recognize that it's true.

Finally, we come to that of failure. This fear is tightly linked to that of judgment. We hate to fail, and changing things increases our risk of failure. Who wants to look like a failure? Not me and probably not you. This is a big one. You tried all this before, and it just never stuck. You failed. You felt stupid, weak, and indeed a failure. This is a well-founded and appropriate fear. Failure can have significant and damaging psychological consequences.

Fear is a really significant barrier to change and for good reason. We are talking about survival. This is a core psychological driver in the brain. It is entirely rational and should not be underestimated. But that's not a reason not to change. Fear is a feeling, and feelings can be altered.

What do you do? Simple. Take all of the above into account. Then make sure you come up with a plan for how you are going to actively address these fears. The solution is not to avoid change but rather set realistic and achievable goals. Make your plans' steps small. One small success leading to another.

JUDGMENT

Judgment plays an enormous part in most of our lives. We are weaned on judgment. I'm not blaming our caregivers; it's just the way it is. The reality is that we grow up with hardwired circuits in our brains that lead to us making judgments.

Some judgments are very helpful and indeed critical to survival. These involve assessing risks and threats to our well-being. Not putting your hand in the fire, being wary of strangers, choosing not to take on an adversary alone, or indeed even placing yourself in a situation where you might need to do so are all helpful judgments.

But we have to be careful and mindful, as some judgments are potentially very damaging. These judgments typically concern our opinions of others. If individuals don't fit our brain's view of the world, then we judge them, often in a poor way. They are a threat to our understanding of what is "right." They threaten our reality. This is understandable behavior to a certain extent, as they are probably from a different tribe. However, we need to be careful not to be casually dismissive of them or their opinions because they may well have something to teach us. And remember, change requires an open mind—the willingness to entertain and generate new attitudes and core beliefs. Learning to accept others helps us accept our new self.

This leads me to perhaps the greatest fear: judgment about you. So much of what we do in life is driven by our concern with this issue of judgment directed at us. If you think about it, a great deal of your anxiety is about fear of being judged. Now you understand the cause of this fear: being judged as *different* risks rejection and being ostracized.

Self-judgment often leads to fear of failure. Judgment is like a voice in your head. I often ask patients if they've ever thought about whose voice it really is. It probably belongs to your mother, your father, or some other significant caregiver, including teachers—or, in reality, a combination of all these people. It's important to understand this because once you recognize and understand its presence and significance, you can actively address it.

Clearly a powerful barrier to success in personal growth and change is judgment, so we need a plan to overcome it. I don't mean get rid of it; that's probably almost impossible and definitely dangerous. To survive and be successful, you need to develop an awareness of judgment and its appropriateness in a given situation. But you also need to develop strategies to deal with it.

AND WE'RE BACK TO PLANS!

The way to deal with these barriers to change are going to sound very familiar: identify the problem; create the plan; write the plan down. Take action and carry out the plan. While carrying out the plan, check in on a regular basis (Me-Time) and ask two simple questions: "Are we on plan, and is the plan still relevant?"

In this case, the goal is how to address these feelings and fears. For example, for many people, the fear is judgment that they are just not good enough. The parental voice ringing in their heads tells them, "You could do better. You don't try hard enough. You should be like your brother. He's so helpful, and he's always near the top of the class."

This voice loses the initial person's identity over time and becomes your own: "I am not good enough. I could do better. My brother is so much more successful."

I see this even in people at the top of their game. They think they're still not good enough, and they're still striving to please that voice. It's often the case that in reality the brother is on his fourth career and second meaningful relationship. His life is no less chaotic.

Why is this important and mentioned here? Because if subconsciously you feel you are not good enough, then any change that might end up in failure is a real threat to your mental well-being and thus best avoided. This leads you to accept the current situation over the potential benefits derived from altering your life.

The goal: develop a realistic view of yourself on a daily basis and silence the critical voice of judgment.

The motivation: An ability to be satisfied with yourself. A determination to feel good and to accept that failure is neither a sign of failure as a human nor the end of the world. Feeling that you are good enough allows you to more easily accept the inevitable judgments and failures that will confront you.

The plan:

Take inventory of what my life is actually like. List my successes as well as failures. You will recognize that there are typically many more successes than failures, and as you get older, the spread between the two usually becomes larger with the passage of time. Make a list of the triggers that precipitate the feeling of "I'm not good enough."

Write down who the voice really belongs to: a caregiver perhaps, or a teacher?

Develop a strategy to address the feeling and fear when it arises. Perhaps put a list of your successes on your phone and actively review the list before starting a meeting, commencing a project, or when you're feeling down about yourself

Remember, it's the doing that matters. The writing down of a list of successes clarifies your thoughts, and reading that list brings you back to reality. These actions, not thoughts, are what rewire those circuits in your brain. Ultimately, the fear of judgment is a feeling. You can learn to sit with feelings however uncomfortable. What you have achieved in life is fact. This is what matters! This is reality.

Then evaluate: Are your attitudes and beliefs beginning to shift? Do you feel better about yourself? Can you make some small changes without deep anxiety? Are you beginning to manage the feeling and achieve your desired outcome?

Your Mindset Is Your Choice—and Only You Can Change It

Many people already know that how they live is probably not healthy. Most understand that what you eat influences your health. We have been told that we need to take exercise and sleep more. So if we know all of this, then why don't we just change? Why do we find it so challenging to transform our lives in a meaningful way?

In addition to the barriers to change as previously mentioned, there are lots of other reasons, and I will review the critical ones here.

First is that we discount future risk over the present reward. In other words, we will take today's pleasure knowing that it is not necessarily good for us and indeed may well harm us in the future because our brain subconsciously and sometimes consciously ignores the future risk.

Second, we tend to accept a lower reward if it is immediate rather than a greater reward in the future. This is why we gravitate toward instant gratification. Most people will take the $100 today rather than wait for a $2,000 payout next year. There are several psychological reasons for this, and many of them are both understandable and possibly even beneficial in the immediate time frame. Unfortunately, this strategy often doesn't serve you well in the long run.

The third reason is that you perceive your current life as comfortable even if it's not going quite right. It's the shoe that fits, even if it's not the right shoe for the job or it's developed a hole in the sole.

Fourth, we are inherently "lazy." From a biological viewpoint, our ecosystem is energy-expenditure conscious. As an organism, we have a natural tendency to do just enough to survive and no more. Change takes effort.

Last, we absolutely don't like to be uncomfortable, even for a short while. We spend a great deal of time doing everything we can to avoid any form of discomfort.

Who wants to give up sugar, stop drinking alcohol, eat a healthy, "boring" diet, and suffer through the discomfort of exercise? Miss out on the late-night TV show? Who wants to be hungry? Who wants to stop having fun?

The fundamental challenge to change is our mindset and the stories we create in our heads. Some of this is conscious, but a great deal more is simply basic psychology, indeed primitive psychology. We are wired not to change, and, more importantly, we are wired not to be different.

Mindset is an important component to change. It's critical to understand that how and what you think shapes your attitudes and behaviors.

Think about all those broken New Year resolutions that you never started on day one or, more typically, you failed to keep after the first week. What's that about? It's not like you're stupid or ignorant. You know what is unhelpful in your life. You have great intentions, but you're only human, right? Next week, next month, no, next year. "It's Mary's birthday next week anyway, and I'll be forty next year. Let's start then." Sound familiar? The never-ending cycle of procrastination, inactivity, and disappointment, perhaps even guilt.

So what is helpful? The answer is actually quite straightforward: you need to learn and develop the skills to take control of your life. Literally, *you can choose.*

Most of the time, we feel that our life is out of our control. It's an absolute truth that a lot of what happens around us is indeed outside our control. The secret is to accept that truth and make the changes within the life you lead rather than trying to change the world around you.

In reality, you can control only two things: how you think and how you behave. For many people, even controlling how they think and act is challenging. The good news is that we can change through learned practices and acquiring new skillsets, which produce new attitudes.

At very basic levels, you can choose how you get to your office. You can decide to walk up the stairs, which takes minimal effort and a couple of minutes longer rather than riding the elevator. Parking your car in the furthest parking spot at the grocery store and walking a little further rather than fighting over the nearest empty space is similarly your choice.

The challenge, of course, is that much of what we do is subconscious, and thus we are completely unaware not only of why we made a choice but that we made a choice at all. Understanding this allows you to recognize that you need to consciously change your behaviors. This is part of mindfulness: being aware and paying attention.

Once you become more aware, you can take positive steps to change the way you think about things and, along with new learned behaviors, rewire your subconscious brain. Just like learning a new language, sport, or any skill, conscious effort and practice leads to automatic behavior.

This includes both thoughts and actions. Think about learning to drive: it was so difficult at the beginning, but after a few hundred hours behind the wheel, it became totally automatic, carried out unconsciously. It is now so automatic that you get in the car, chat to your passenger, and arrive at your destination. Chances are that you will remember nothing about the route and absolutely nothing about how you drove the car.

So when you say you cannot change, you can. First, it takes a decision to do so, and then it takes practice.

Critical to this, however, as I have mentioned several times previously, is a genuine and deep desire to change. Without this you are probably doomed to failure because change is hard work; it takes time and commitment.

THE NEUROSCIENCE OF CHANGE

But how does this change happen?

Our brain is made up of 86 billion nerve cells called neurons. Surrounding them is a matrix of supporting cells called glial or glue cells. These glue cells turn out to be as important as the nerve cells themselves. Astrocytes and oligodendrocytes along with microglia cells keep the brain's networks working in a controlled and coordinated fashion as one unit. Individual cells are connected in a complex of webs and pathways, which neuroscientists have mapped with remarkable accuracy. Everything that we do is controlled by activations of multiple networks.

As I have mentioned before, the more you use a network, the stronger that network's links become, and the easier it is for your mind to go there. These strong networks are called highways and give rise to our unique behavior patterns and habits.

For example, our personalities are a mix of genetics, habits, and early-life experiences all encoded in these dominant highways. The way we react to certain situations is programmed into our brain. How often do you blurt something out, laugh, or become angry without even thinking about it? The answer is most of the time.

Your reactions and interactions are mostly preprogrammed by the way in which these circuits developed during your time in your mother's womb, your childhood, and early adult experiences. Your life story shapes your brain highways and makes you who you are. It's not only your thoughts and actions that are programmed but also your response to painful stimuli, giving rise to the different pain experiences that we all recognize. Some people really do have high pain thresholds, just as some have low tolerance to pain. Lastly, we now recognize that this extends to the entire neuro-immune system. So what happens to you in the early part of your life programs your body and its response to all sorts of challenges.

Many neural networks are developed in response to your childhood environment, both physical and emotional. Further, our selective perception bias reinforces these circuits, so sad people's brains search out sad data and block happy information, while optimistic people do the opposite. The older you are, the more reinforced the highways, and the more challenging it becomes to change.

The good news is that you can change the wiring and the structure of the networks. Old highways can be put into disuse, and new ones can be built. Our central nervous system exhibits something called plasticity. This means that it is pliable and can change its physical structure and its circuits.

The idea that we get one set of nerve cells as a child is false. We create new neurons while removing old and worn-out ones all the time. We even prune the side branches of individual neurons that make connections with other neurons, and indeed build new branches creating new connections. This is why the more we use a particular highway or network, the stronger it becomes. It's equally true if you don't use a particular network, the connections are pruned, and the pathway becomes weaker. It's just like going to the gym: if you work a particular group of muscles, they get stronger; if you neglect another group, they get weaker.

· ·

This is not a casual analogy because, as I have noted before, taking regular physical exercise enhances this process of remodeling neuronal circuits in the brain.

· ·

As I mentioned previously, my patients tell me all the time that they can't change the way they live. I advise them to question the way they think and consider replacing the words "cannot change" with "cannot be bothered to change," or, more often, "don't really want to change."

I ask them, "Do you think you could learn to drive a car, learn a new language, or play an instrument?" The answer of course is yes. It might be difficult and challenging, particularly as we get older, but we can all do it.

So it's not a matter of whether you *can*; it's a case of really *wanting* to change things. This is about mindset, not ability.

Remember, change itself is a process. It takes time to develop as an idea and mature into a real behavioral modification. Typically, we don't just wake up one day and think, *Hmm, I'm going to be a new person and embrace a new life today*. Well, at least not in a meaningful way. Sure, after a hard night out and suffering from a hangover or waking up feeling bloated and uncomfortable after too much food, everyone is going to get a new life. That's not the same as a real desire to change.

A real desire to refashion your life comes on slowly as you begin to think differently about the way you live. Real change starts with a willingness to move away from your current belief and behavior comfort zones and become a child again, willing to try new things without any critical judgment. That's why kids are so much fun and why they learn so quickly; they are not hampered by fixed ideas and habits. They are not weighed down by fear of judgment. They can be anything they want to be, if not for real, then certainly in their imagination.

Then they act it out, and in their play, they "learn" by rewiring their brain's circuits and networks. It's the doing that changes them. They don't think or talk themselves into new behaviors.

Adults are no different. Quality therapy is based on the idea of letting go again so that you can allow yourself to evolve into someone different from the current you. In a sense, it allows you to be a child at play, willing to make mistakes and accept failures.

STAGES OF CHANGE

The first step in making lasting alterations is a recognition that you want to feel different and live a better life. This is the beginning of a longer process that actually takes months to unfold. That's okay because you are looking for permanent lifestyle modifications that are sustainable. This week's latest fad may satisfy the human mind's need for novelty, which is of course why fads are so pervasive and common in society, but on the whole, fads do not lead to permanent and meaningful change.

Failure to recognize that remodeling a life is a process that will unravel over time is one of the barriers to change. The take-home message here is cut yourself some slack when you fall off the wagon. If you do fall off, you will have to generate a little extra effort to get back up. We all need a break when we are doing something that challenges us, but don't make the break too long because you're just making it too difficult to start again.

Stop worrying about whether you'll be successful, and recognize that you're going through a process. Just keep going by doing.

As a reminder: *precontemplation* is the period of time when we wonder whether we want to do something. It can last for months or longer. If we decide, for whatever reason, that we *do* want change, we then go through a period of more focused *contemplation*. This is the time when we begin to consolidate our thoughts into a more definable idea and indeed plan to change.

Next comes an *action phase* when we actually do something to try to initiate the change. If we are successful, then we go through a period of *consolidation* or maintenance. Finally the change either sticks in some form or not, and the process of change comes to an end.

Make a Plan to Change

Some things are easier to change than others.

A great deal of what we do, say, and feel is automatic. These are subconscious behaviors, thoughts, and feelings, like slouching, sucking in your breath, biting your nails, or being irrationally grumpy with a partner or friend.

Some behaviors and feelings are indulgences, and you do have control over them. They are conscious thoughts and decisions, such as choosing to eat a certain way, practicing safe sex, and going to the gym to train.

Some behaviors are just daily things we need to do: when to eat, when to go to bed, when to leave for work.

All three types of behaviors are slightly different, and all three require a separate approach. But all of them can be modified if you want to change them and are prepared to make an effort. As you develop self-awareness or mindfulness skills with Me-time practice, which will spill over into your daily life, you will be able to spot these behaviors. Once you're aware of them, you can decide to work toward addressing them. For example, noticing yourself slouching leads you to rectify your posture to a better one; recognizing an uncontrolled flash of irritation enables you to ask why and perhaps address the true reason.

You have a goal. You need to break the process of getting there into little steps.

There are a few other things you can do to increase your likelihood of success when making a plan.

FAKE IT TO MAKE IT

As Jordan Peterson suggests in the first chapter of his book *12 Rules for Life*, stand up straight and pull your shoulders back. Be a lobster. You will feel better.

Interestingly, the idea of "fake it to make it" has been around for a long time. Science has caught up with this idea reportedly first promoted by Alcoholics Anonymous.

There are many books out there teaching various techniques to visualize yourself in your dream job, new outfit, super fit, or whatever it is you want to be. The trouble with this is that the evidence suggests that, far from helping, this form of visualization can have negative impacts on your chances of being successful. There is some psychological quirk whereby if we imagine the final product, we put less effort into obtaining it. Simply put, visualization is a potential barrier to achieving your objective. More than that, it sets you up for failure, and failure is a bad strategy to be successful in making meaningful and lasting changes.

It's very important that you understand this: Doing is much more important than thinking. So the strategy to change is not thinking about it—I'll keep banging the drum—it's doing it. Fake it to make it.

Understand the difference between thoughts and actions. Thoughts are random, and holding a single, logical train of thought is difficult. Other thoughts invade all the time; we forget what we were thinking a few thoughts back. Thinking for most people is chaotic; this in turn is distracting.

Thinking about stuff also brings it to mind. When you decide not to do something, you will think about it more. *I'm not going to eat chocolate, smoke, or drink.* The more you go there, all you can think about is chocolate, a cigarette, or a drink. Attempting to suppress thoughts has the same effect. The more you are told not to think about something, the more you think about it. The mind is funny that way. So what's the solution? *Do* something else that keeps your mind occupied.

Try writing things down—action. We can look back and reference what we wrote five lines back. The fascinating and very helpful thing about writing is that it clarifies things. The first thing I teach is to get into the habit of writing things down. Not a daily novel, just short notes, thoughts, and ideas. (Writing this book clarified my often-disjointed thoughts into a clearer set of core beliefs and ideas.)

This applies to everything. Something bad happened? No need to talk it out with friends; just write down your thoughts and concerns. Why was it bad? What were the real consequences? If you do this a couple of times, you will find that how and what you feel about an event will change. Typically, your feelings will change for the better, and almost certainly they will be more rational and objective. Contrast this with the chaos of thoughts.

Try writing down what you are grateful for. This sounds like positive affirmation, but it's not. We know that if you just write down three things that you are grateful for every night before you go to bed, you will be happier.

If you behave like a happy person, we know you will feel like a happy person. Fake it to make it.

FORGET ABOUT LUCK

There is no such thing as being lucky or unlucky. There's plenty of research about this, and the conclusion is straightforward. The reality is we make our own luck.

Don't confuse luck with chance. If you go to a casino, then we are not discussing luck; we are discussing chance. Casinos are all about the odds, which, by the way, are not stacked in your favor. Gambling is a mugs game.

So what makes somebody "lucky" in life? The truth is that lucky people tend to be those without anxiety and fear. Fear narrows our attention and perspective on the world around us. So-called lucky individuals have less fear and anxiety. They have a broader attentional spotlight. In other words, they capture more of life.

People with so-called good luck tend to be flexible, opportunistic, follow their intuition, and are resilient. They see failure as a good thing, a learning opportunity, and not a disaster. They use tough moments in life to empower them, not defeat them. And of course, they make plans.

The brain is interesting: if you tell people that you are lucky in life, they will recall stories that support that belief. If you tell people you are unlucky, then they tend to recall stories that support that belief. We create our own reality. We create the story in our own head by use of words and indeed actions.

To create your own luck, you just have to change the dialogue and create the correct story—the helpful one.

UNDERSTAND THE DIFFERENCE BETWEEN PLEASURE AND HAPPINESS

Psychologists and philosophers have debated the difference between happiness and pleasure for a long time. Neurobiologists and neuro-chemists are trying to track down exactly how it all works. But we can make a few observations that we all recognize. Pleasure does not always lead to happiness. In fact, it seems that the pursuit of too much pleasure leads to a loss of happiness and indeed being unhappy.

Pleasure is felt in various ways, but it's short-lived. It's often an "in your tummy" or all-over, visceral feeling. After the moment is over, we often feel empty inside. Things that cause pleasure include eating, sugar, sex, alcohol, drugs, shopping, gambling, and social media. These are in part driven by a neurotransmitter called dopamine that drives circuits related to anticipation of something "fun" and a reward.

What's important to understand here is that constantly wanting to experience pleasure behaviors has the potential to lead to addictive behavior. Furthermore, too much "wanting of a pleasure experience," rather than too much enjoyment of that experience, can actually lead to unhappiness. Unhappy people often feel that more pleasurable ex-periences, and more intense pleasure will lead to happiness. Actually, the complete opposite occurs. Too much pleasure, and importantly the pursuit or wanting of too much pleasure, leads to unhappiness!

The other thing about pleasure is that when it concerns behaviors that are primarily about me ("selfish"), then it is more likely to lead to unhappiness. When providing pleasurable experiences for others, it's less so.

In general, pleasure is short-lived and is fine in moderate doses, but if abused, it has a negative effect on happiness. We also recognize that too much dopamine appears to inhibit the production of serotonin (see below).

Take-home message: be careful; the pursuit of pleasure does not necessarily lead to happiness. Often pleasure leads to unhappiness.

Happiness is different from pleasure. It has different neurotransmitters. One is serotonin. This is associated with feelings of calm, focus, and of course happiness. Most of our serotonin in the body is found and produced in the gut. Yet again, we close a loop. Gut health is linked to happiness and well-being. Happiness and indeed its sibling contentedness are more of a state of being rather than a feeling. When you are happy or content, you just are right with the world.

So in summary, pleasure is often short-lived, empty, and can lead to a desire for more. Happiness on the other hand is a longer lasting feeling of calmness, of being at peace with yourself and the world around you.

Being happy matters. Being unhappy is associated with increased illness and poorer quality of life. The opposite is true: being happy leads to a longer, healthier, and more fulfilling life. Most important, happiness does not necessarily come from success; it actually causes it!

Does having money and possessions make you happy? No! Not having enough money to meet basic needs in your particular environment is associated with lower levels of happiness. However, once you have enough to meet these universal and basic requirements, having more does not necessarily make you happier. In fact, there is some evidence to support the opposite.

Psychologists have demonstrated that buying experiences rather than stuff makes you happier, and for longer. Buying stuff for other people has the same effect.

Psychologists have also clearly shown that we like variety and things that challenge us, like learning a new skill or taking up a new hobby.

How about challenging yourself to be healthier and then learning how to do it? There's lots of variety and challenges here, along with new experiences and new knowledge. After reading this book, you're already well on your way!

So how can you be happy? Yes, you got it, by doing things! Certain behaviors also stimulate happiness. I like to call them the five Cs:

1. **Communication.** Eye to eye, in person allowing for mirroring and thus empathy. (Social media is the antithesis: pleasure, "alone together," isolation, and depression.)

2. **Connection.** Vital. We need to be part of a family/tribe/clan. Don't forget hugs!

3. **Contribution.** Altruism. Giving or doing something for others for the sake of giving, not for recognition.

4. **Cope.** Exercise, sleep, Me-Time (mindfulness), stress management.

5. **Cook.** In a group or partnership, real food, mainly plants. Cooking this way requires Communication, Connection, and Contribution.

Your To-Do List

- Take control of your life. Literally, you can choose.

- Become a *doer* not just a *thinker*. Doing changes you; thinking does not.

    - Visualization of you at the end of the journey—slim, successful, perfect life, etc.—is not helpful.

        - Visualization of the steps that you are going to take to get to slim, successful, and a better life is helpful.

- Get a diary and write in it. Writing helps clarify your storyline. It helps rewire the brain.

- Work at ditching fear. Fear of failure, fear of judgment, fear of change.

    - Stop imagining unrealistic goals. You're setting yourself up for failure, and this is a significant barrier to change.

    - Cut yourself some slack to make mistakes. Fail sometimes and make a fool of yourself. (Who cares?)

    - Anticipate success but accept failure. Persevere.

    - When things go wrong, don't beat yourself up; just learn from it.

    - Perfection is the enemy of success.

- Get a new clan or create your own. Choose people who are like you want to be.

- Choose a mentor. Who do you really admire? How do they live their life?

- Put the rock down. Stop carrying old worries and distresses with you. Life moved on. Leave your past behind.

Are you ready to make a change? Yeah, you are!

Get out that plan and everything you've written down thus far. It's time to bring it all together.

CHAPTER 9

PUTTING IT ALL TOGETHER

· ·

A journey is made up of individual parts.

If I want to get to London, I start by walking to my car, a series of individual steps. Goal number one accomplished.

Then I drive to the station via a specific route. Goal number two accomplished.

Then I make another series of individual steps, which take me to the train and so forth.

For those of us who have been traveling a specific route for a long time, this journey is easy. It may be boring and tedious sometimes, but it is certainly not frightening.

But if you've never traveled a long distance before, or it's a new trip to a novel destination, it can all seem very daunting. However, the solution is simple: we just need to break it into steps.

One Step at a Time

To be successful in making the changes you want, there are some simple, practical steps that have been shown to be effective by psychological research.

In fact, the key has already been mentioned: take your larger goal (the long, arduous journey) and break it into smaller steps. Suddenly, it becomes manageable. When you recognize this simple truth and form the plan of how you are going to do it, the task becomes much less daunting. More importantly, you're going to be successful. Completion of each sub-part of your plan builds confidence to move to the next stage. And suddenly you're there!

Get out your plan from Chapter 1. Let's review it and break it down.

The first step is to define your goals. You need to be specific about these. For example:

- I want to be able to run a 5K in thirty minutes.

- I want to lose five pounds in the next two months.

- I want to go to bed by eleven o'clock six days out of the week.

Note that these are all very clearly defined.

The next step is to write down your deeply felt, personal reason for having the goal. Remember this is *your* own motivation, not someone else's idea or advice. It's why *you* want to go through the process. This is critical to success because when the doing gets tough, this is where you remind yourself why you started the project.

The final step is to create a plan for each goal. The best way to do this is to decide four to five steps that will get you there. Again, you need to be specific. What are you going to do? When are you going to do it? How long is it going to take?

Write down these steps. This is where you need to be realistic, so put some thought into it. This is the first doing event: moving thought onto paper.

Let's look at the example of significantly reducing sugar in your diet—something we all need to aspire to. There are two ways of doing this: suddenly or slowly. It doesn't really matter which way you choose, but you need to set the goal and a timeline for achieving that goal.

- Goal: Remove all added sugar from my diet in four weeks.

- Why: Because I recognize eating sugar makes me feel tired, hungry, and grumpy about an hour after I have eaten it.

- Plan:

  - Step 1: In the first week, I'm going to remove chocolate and ice cream.

  - Step 2: In the second week, I'm going to take time to cook three evening meals rather than eating premade/processed meals that contain added sugars.

  - Step 3: I'm going to stop adding sugar to my tea or coffee.

  - Step 4: I'm going to cut out all cookies, cakes, candies, and sweets.

  - Step 5: I am going to stop buying sugars to keep in the house.

Last, I would suggest that you set a reward for achieving your goals. This is totally legitimate and a great motivator for many people.

- When I achieve this, I'm going to reward myself by taking my partner out to dinner, treating us both to a great meal, including dessert!

The important thing about all of this is to be realistic.

The other thing to note is that there is no mention of "losing weight" or feeling better; these are goals, not steps to get there. You know that this will benefit you, period, so you don't need to fantasize about it. Just set the goal, write down the steps, and then—you guessed it—just follow the plan.

Okay, I think you understand the message. Change is a doing thing, and to be successful, you need a plan of action to get you where you want to be.

Now a couple of philosophical things to bear in mind.

Life Is Just Plain Difficult

Life is just plain difficult. This is a simple truth, and it was the conclusion of one of the world's greatest philosophers and the father of modern psychology, Siddhartha Gautama, also known as the Buddha. It was a view also shared by the philosophical school of Stoicism. Both these separate schools have provided the foundation for several modern psychological treatment strategies including CBT, DBT, mindfulness, and acceptance therapies. The application of their basic understanding of the nature of our lives can be used as an important tool in addressing all of our health challenges and aspirations. We can take two main themes from their many insights.

The first observation was that life is inherently filled with "suffering." Translated into today's terms, this means that it is complicated, messy, uncomfortable, and difficult…even when going well. Too much fun and too many possessions have downsides, just as much as having too little or no fun at all. Underpinning this suffering is our mortality—an uncomfortable truth that many of us try to deny.

If we stop to think about it, we know this is true! Life is just inherently complicated, difficult, and sometimes very painful, just as it can have moments of great joy and happiness.

The second observation was that we have a way of making this situation worse. We spend most of our lives pretending it is not true. Much of what we do is an attempt to create buffers that are supposed to prevent us from suffering, but this is ultimately an exercise in futility.

We also increase our distress with our multiple desires. In the material world, we want more money, a nicer car, the bigger house, better vacations, better relationships, friends, career success, and more. On a personal basis, we desire to be individuals who are respected by others. We want and expect happiness, love, freedom from illness, a life without sadness, a life without difficulty, and ultimately we all wish we can avoid death and the departure from this world of our loved ones, friends, and of course ourselves.

If you reflect on your life, a lot of your "difficulties" are because you want some parts, or indeed all parts, of it to be different. Unfortunately, many of us deal with this problem in a multitude of often unhealthy ways. We spend so much of our life trying to mold reality and the world around us to make it comfortable rather than accepting it the way it is. So much physical and emotional energy is expended in futile efforts to protect ourselves, rather than trying to find something to be content with in the moment that we are in.

Added to this, we make life more uncomfortable because we fill it with judgment. We start with self, then we turn to others, and then our surroundings. If you contemplate your internal dialogue, ask yourself, "How often am I judgmental?" The scary answer is most of the time. "I should be better at this or that; I should have done this or that." "Why am I so lazy, fat, unfit?" "Why are they Christians, gay, cliquish, vegetarians—aka, different from me?" Finally, "This is a messy home, dirty neighborhood, terrible government, bad country." And so we go.

Working toward being less judgmental is a sensible and helpful goal. It will bring you some peace and go a long way to reducing your discomfort with life.

Last, your day-to-day level of frustration is directly related to the distance you choose to place between reality, the actual current situation you find yourself in, and your expectations of what you desire or wanted it to be. The further apart from reality you place your expectations and even aspirations, the more frustrated you will be. Of course a small gap is beneficial as it can motivate. But beyond that, the only product of a wide disparity is increasing frustration, and the natural product of this is stress and distress.

Understand these separate but related truths: life is naturally difficult, and unrealistic expectations and judgment lead to stress. Deciding to accept them as truths and then live accordingly, although challenging, has the potential for enormous gains in overall health and well-being.

Accepting that life is difficult and complicated, and that we cannot change this fact, leads to significant reductions in stress. Couple this with a realistic set of *aspirations of what might be* rather than *expectations of what should be*, and you will be well on your way to improving your quality of life.

Realistic Goals

If you have reached this point by reading the whole book, well done. That's a lot of information and ideas that are not always easy to follow or recall. (If you have jumped here, that's fine, too.)

What you should take away is a simple concept: to be healthy and diminish your risk of becoming physically and mentally unwell, you need to take a holistic approach to health. Everything you think, speak, and do has an effect on every part of your body. What you eat, whether you move and take exercise, the amount and quality of your sleep, and your strategies for minimizing stress and strain on your body and mind governs who you are.

So you want to change the way you live, a little and maybe a lot? We explored some of the barriers to change and how you might get to your chosen goal. There are lots of natural blocks to changing; they're all very real and entirely understandable. But once you appreciate this, then the way forward is much easier.

So let's put it all together. The secret to success is first asking some questions.

Where are you trying to get to? What is your goal? It sounds silly and obvious, but I am constantly talking to patients who don't have a clear idea where they want to be in one year, five years, and so on. Most of us don't typically get in a car and just head off somewhere; we have a destination. If we don't, we feel uneasy. If you don't have a clear idea where you are heading, or a goal, you are setting yourself up for failure, which has significant negative psychological consequences for most people.

Just as important is **Why** do you want to get there? This one is easier, but people typically get it wrong. They think they should change because other people tell them they should. That is very unhelpful. You change because you want to. If you don't want to change deep in your soul, then you're not going to.

Finally, **What** is your plan?

So there we have it. Let's set an example of a realistic aspiration. It may not happen, but you are going to give your best effort by actually doing it.

Where: I want to lose ten pounds. (I'm going to suggest you start with five pounds—and certainly NOT "I want to lose forty pounds by next month." Set realistic goals, remember? Once successful, you can set a new one.)

Then ask **Why?** I want to be ten pounds lighter because I hate feeling short of breath when I bend over to tie my shoelaces. (You choose the reason, and in reality you probably have several. Make sure that you choose things that really matter to **you**. Not, "I want to lose ten pounds because my mother said I look overweight," or "My doctor told me I need to lose weight." The question is what motivates you deep down inside? If the answer is nothing, then I'm going to suggest that you will struggle to succeed. Honestly you are probably going to fail with all the negative consequences.)

Finally, **What** is the plan?

1. I am going to set a goal of removing all added sugar and starches from my diet for two weeks and see if I might lose three pounds. Then I am going to set a new aspiration and a new plan.

2. I am going to remove all sugar and starches from the kitchen and my shopping list.

3. I am going to plan a menu for two weeks.

4. I am going to think about the pitfalls and traps and make a separate plan for those. For example, "It's Auntie Bertha's birthday on Tuesday, and I love cake." Or "It's parents' night on Thursday, and there are always sodas, cookies, and cakes there." (What are your plans to deal with these events?)

Next, write the goal, the whys, and the plan down on a piece of paper and stick it on the fridge.

You are ready to make a lasting change!

Tracking Your Health: Wellness "Scores"

We covered Me-Time earlier as a way of monitoring your progress. I mentioned that it is always helpful to keep a record and write things down. Recall the four questions: how do I feel emotionally, mentally, physically, and why?

It's worth going a little further and tracking your overall Wellness "Score."

There are many different "scores" out there, but here is my *how to take stock* worksheet. Remember both physical and mental or psychological well-being matter.

Most of this checklist is done by you, but there are a couple of basic lab tests that will require a health professional to request.

Think about your answers and jot down some notes. This is not a comprehensive medical questionnaire, but it's quite sufficient to assess your overall health. It covers the important markers. (Note cholesterol is not on the list.)

What to do with the answers? Compare them with the goals that you decided on. Are you actually doing something to reach them, and can you see the results? Again, be patient. The important thing is that you now have a written record, and you can track your progress.

In reality, there are an increasing number of sophisticated apps to help both assess and track your health, and more apps are on the way. Technology is going to transform the way you monitor your physical and mental well-being along with your progress at home without any medical intervention. Indeed, that's the point: tracking your own health with the goal to keep you away from sickness care providers. Just ensure that, as a minimum, these parameters are being measured.

PERSONAL HEALTH ASSESSMENT

Most of this checklist is done by you, but there are a couple of basic lab tests that will require a health professional to request.

Mental/Emotional

	Healthy/Change/Unhealthy
Are you content with your overall life?	Y/N
Are you in a fulfilling relationship or content to be single if not?	Y/N
Do you have a group of friends and acquaintances that support you?	Y/N
Are you clear headed or foggy brained?	Clear/Foggy

Complete the Patient Health Questionnaire (PHQ-9) and Generalized Anxiety Disorder Questionaire (GAD-7) Both are widely available online with automatic scoring.

Depressed	Y/N
Anxious	Y/N

Physical

	Healthy/Change/Unhealthy
What is your height and weight? BMI?	<24/24-30/>30
What is your abdominal circumference at the tummy button?*	<37/37-40/>40 M <33/33-36/>36 F
What is your blood pressure?	<120/80, 120/80-140/100, >140/100
What is your resting pulse rate?	<70, 70-90, >90
What is your HbA1C%? (health practitioner to measure) Measure of your average blood sugar.	<5.7, 5.7-6.4, >6.4
What is your CRP (best) or ESR? (health practitioner to measure)	<2/2-10/ >10
What is your vitamin D level? (health practitioner to measure) *Should be > 50 - <100 ng/ml*	50-100, 50-30, <30
How many flights of stairs can you walk nonstop without being short of breath?	>4/1-4/<1

Lifestyle

	Healthy/Change/Unhealthy
How much of your diet is junk food?	<20%/20-60%/>60%
Do you consume sugary drinks?	Y/N
Do you exercise 5 times per week?	Y/N
How many hours do you sleep?	7-8, <7, <6
Do you have a stress management plan?	Y/N

*(I'm being kind)

CONCLUSION

By today's standards, my grandfather was a quack. In reality, he was a highly trained physician, surgeon, and—as it happens—a veterinary doctor.

His apparent challenge was that he lived before the arrival of modern pharmacology and Big Pharma. His only tools as a very skilled practitioner were what we now consider to be alternative therapies. There were almost no medications worth talking about during 1910 to 1935. Certainly nothing comparable to the complex pharmacopeias available today.

He practiced the fast-disappearing art of medicine. It required empathy and understanding, along with validation of people and their stories. With a solid grounding in common-sense psychology, along with a pragmatic approach to his patients and their problems, he understood that a person's environment was critical to good health. He understood the importance of a supportive social network and family, clean air and sunshine, adequate rest, and good nutrition. Most important of all, he looked after people, not diseases or conditions.

The fascinating thing is that, by all accounts, his patients did very well. Even though he did not have access to antibiotics or any other medications worth talking about, they did not all die from infections or other chronic diseases, such as high blood pressure or diabetes. They were on the whole a fairly healthy group of people, and the majority lived long, productive lives.

My Influences

I've seen the same outcome in another place, too.

In one of my jobs, I came into contact with a group of fit and well elderly individuals. They live in a remote location and only gained access to electricity about thirty-five years ago. Most of them easily make it into their eighties and nineties. Several are over a hundred years of age with clear, sharp minds.

What did these people have in common? They all ate modest amounts because there was not a lot of food. The food they had was fresh and, on the whole, locally grown. They cooked it.

They walked everywhere because cars were nonexistent. Exercise was just part of a typical, day-to-day life. Nobody went to a gym.

They slept long hours because there was no television. Sunset meant it was time to quiet down and get ready for bed. Natural, not artificial, light dictated the structure of their life.

They had a lot more downtime. Their life was challenging and a struggle, but they were resilient. They did not have time for emotional drama. They had realistic aspirations of what life was and how it would be. They were, by today's standards, modest in their desires.

They interacted more with each other. They lived in communities, practiced the art of conversation, and contributed to each other's lives.

These are the attributes found in the so-called blue zones, places on earth where people live long and healthy lives.

As you can probably tell, my grandfather and these people had a significant influence on my thinking. Why? Because, in short, the results—long, healthy lives—speak louder than all the theory flowing around.

The Simple Message

The message is simplicity in itself. Health does not come out of a pill bottle or a hospital. It does not come from a doctor's surgery or clinic. Health comes from within; it comes from you. It's about how you were born and then nurtured. It's about your childhood experience and subsequent life story. It's about your internal neurological wiring and the structure of your immune system, your neuro-immune system. It's based upon how these two systems are intertwined and tuned. Ultimately it depends upon how you choose to live and experience your life. The story you choose to create in your mind.

But you are not alone in this world, and so as I draw to a close, I would like to leave you with a couple of final key thoughts.

Cooperation in a Complex System

I want to upend the long-held theory that success is based upon survival of the fittest. This is not necessarily true in evolution and certainly not in ecology.

In reality, successful ecosystems, like successful societies and businesses, are based on cooperation and cooperative behavior. This whole book is about this simple truth.

The human body is the pinnacle of the evolution of cooperation in a single organism. Our body consists of approximately thirty-five trillion cells. There are about two hundred classes of very diverse specialist human cells, which can survive only because they work together cooperatively. None can live without the others.

Depending upon where you live, this cooperation extends to a community of between 3,000 and 7,000 species of bacteria that are present in the human body. This colony outnumbers human cells at 60–100 trillion. This is not to mention the fungi, archaea, viruses, protozoa, mites, and worms that contribute to the entire ecosystem that is your body.

Although this may be a disquieting thought to many, it's a fact. This group of diverse human cells and companion organisms are obliged to exist in balance and harmony inside us—a meta-organism, an ecosystem on the move. This cooperative harmony is key to being and remaining healthy and well.

Thinking of the body as a dynamic ecosystem can help you understand health (and sickness) more comprehensively.

Along these lines, the medical and healing communities are slowly rediscovering an appreciation of the complex interplay among the various cells and organ systems in the body. For a long time, western medicine segregated cardiology (heart), neurology (nerves and the brain), gastroenterology (gut and liver), etc. as if they existed in isolation from each other.

Most damaging, it separated mind from body as if they were somehow existing in isolated spaces. In reality, they are all intimately connected not only physically, but through an exquisitely complex communication network run by the neuro-immune and neuro-endocrine systems of the body.

If anything goes wrong anywhere, it affects every other system, indeed every other cell. This happens in seconds and minutes, as well as over hours, days, and years. This is why it is crucial to have a holistic and integrative approach to both achieving health and wellness, in addition to treating illness.

It remains a common pitfall for many practitioners and patients to attempt to address illness by treating the individual parts, or from their personal perspective. This is in part because of increasing complexity of medical treatments and the need for specialist training. But this type of approach often fails because we must address the problem from a broader perspective.

Health and wellness, and indeed freedom from illness, encompass all aspects of the human experience. The WHO defines health as "the state of complete physical, mental, and social well-being, which is marked not only by the absence of disease or infirmity." Within this definition, health and well-being are intertwined and founded on an individual's subjective perspective on his or her physical, psychological, and social state of being.

To achieve the goal of universal health requires a different approach, one that is inclusive of all members of society. It suggests that if we are to be healthy as individuals, we need to be healthy as a human community. We need to balance our own societal ecosystem. And equally important, we need to relearn how to exist in a cooperative fashion with our environment, the natural world that supports and nourishes us. Just as the final cell in your big toe requires every other cell in the body to be healthy, and the entire human body ecosystem to be in balance to allow it to survive, so do we, as human beings, depend upon our entire environment to be the same.

This book is about just that—balance produced by cooperative behaviors and interactions among unbelievably diverse cells and microorganisms. It is a book about tolerance and cooperation based upon recognition that as much as cells and systems within the body might have different priorities, there needs to be negotiation and compromise to maintain the peace and thus well-being of all.

Nobody is surprised at the consequences of dripping chemicals into an environment slowly over ten years—the slow poisoning of the local ecosystem and the appearance of distorted and stunted plants and diseased animals. Yet we remain perplexed at the fact that after years of stressing and poisoning our bodies, they become sick and fail us.

I have spent literally a lifetime studying this amazing ecosystem both in sickness and in health, and it is beyond wonderment when you glimpse the complexity and unimaginable intricacy of not only each cell, but how they interact together to produce the whole, benefiting every member of the "society" that makes us who we are. The amazing thing to me is that if you take the pressures off, if you provide space for your body to recover by living a balanced life, it almost always will heal and repair itself, returning to a healthy state.

> On the whole, when placed into a healthy environment and fed the correct food, the human body is the master of this type of existence.

However bad the damage, there is always room to regain some health. For many of us, we can regain it completely.

Healthspan versus Lifespan

How you feel during your life is what matters. We all worry about the length of our lives, but I'm going to suggest that it's more appropriate to be concerned about the *quality* of that life: the time you spend being healthy—your healthspan.

Our lifespan has not increased very much. Modern human beings have been reaching three score years and ten (seventy years) for probably well over five thousand years, now eighty to ninety in most developed countries.

However some regions show significant gains on healthspan. For example, in Sweden, the period of life spent in good health is seventy-three for both sexes, about ten years short of the average lifespan. Interestingly, although women do tend to live longer, men enjoy a more extended period of good health in many countries. For example, women in the UK live about 3.5 years longer than men, but the upper limit of good health is 63.4 years, while it's sixty-four years for men. This is very much in line with the World Health Organization's average of 63.5 for the world. In the UK, that translates into twenty years spent with health problems, 24 percent of a life as compared to Sweden, where it represents only 12 percent! That's a significant difference—ten years is a very long time.

It's a complicated subject, but the data show that countries and societies investing in healthy living reap the rewards. Scandinavian countries and Japan enjoy some of the most extended health and lifespans. This is attributed to their philosophy of balance and moderation in everything.

The debate about which lifestyles are associated with the lowest levels of illness and the best quality of life continues. The answer is found in the so-called blue zones of the world. In these communities, people not only live longer, but they live longer in good health. These societies demonstrate all of the Five Elements discussed in this book. They eat real food and in modest amounts. They exercise as part of their daily living, not necessarily as some special, isolated event. (There are exceptions like the widespread practice of daily community exercises, such as tai chi in China.) They practice good sleep habits, and they make time available for themselves while living in communities that excel in cooperative behavior. All of this leads to significant reductions in stress levels. These practices reduce chronic inflammation, which is the root cause of almost all the diseases of aging.

While the debate rages on in the scientific community, and specialist groups market their own biased agendas, we need a common-sense approach. We need to take heed of this simple formula. It's as ancient as humanity.

Good diet, regular exercise and movement, appropriate sleep, some self-reflection, and stress and strain management through realistic aspirations and community living are proven to lead to long, healthy lives.

One of the key goals of working through the ideas in this book is to try to get your healthspan as close to your lifespan as possible, and to extend that lifespan as well. Aiming for ninety to one hundred years mostly in good health is the potential prize; it's the ultimate goal.

Simplicity Is the Key

So there we have it. It really is very straightforward. To move toward better health, you don't have to make massive or radical changes to your life. You just need to start taking some small steps in the five areas outlined in the preceding pages.

So many people are put off by the feeling that it's all too much or too difficult. Change is scary, so approach it in a stepwise fashion rather than through some crazy, dramatic, life-altering New Year's—resolution style.

First, have faith that you can be a different you. You can be well. You can lose weight if you want to, or climb a mountain. Really, you just have to want to do it.

This book took five years to write. It had false starts, and sometimes it sat idle on my computer, but then one day, I decided to finish it. How? By making it a priority in my life.

I made a commitment to myself to share all this knowledge I had shared with others on an individual basis. I made a plan. I sought people who could help me. I joined that clan, and they held me accountable. Then I did something else. I sat down every day and almost without fail wrote a minimum of 250 words per day for four months. That's it. There are more words than that on this page.

One step at a time; one day at a time.

The job was done.

I made it, and I hope you enjoy the outcome. I also hope it helps you find a healthier and happier way to live.

RECOMMENDED READING

Omnivores Dilemma. Michael Pollan

The Healing Power of Mindfulness. Jon Kabat-Zinn

Meditation Is Not What You Think. Jon Kabat-Zinn

Why We Sleep. Matthew Walker

When the Body Says No: The Cost of Hidden Stress. Gabor Maté

In the Realm of Hungry Ghosts. Gabor Maté

12 Rules for Life. Jordan Peterson

Beyond Order. Jordan Peterson

The Dialectical Behavioral Therapy Skills Workbook. Jeffrey Brantley, Jeffrey C. Wood, and Matthew McKay

ACKNOWLEDGMENTS

Writing this book was one of the most challenging things I attempted in my life, and it would never have been completed without the support of so many.

First, I want to thank my staff and colleagues who over the years supported me in my vision of building an integrative approach to assisting patients. With their hard work and commitment, we have been successful.

Second, I would like to acknowledge the many thousands of patients who trusted me and allowed me to guide them. No greater privilege can be given to another. Thank you.

Thank you to my beta readers who kindly worked their way through the first drafts so diligently and whose feedback was critical to shaping this book. Nick, my brother, the only person who I am aware read this book twice. Declan, Jo, Patrick, Sara, Wyn, Nish, and Meghan, thank you all. And Marika, who taught me how to keep fit intelligently while offering good insight into my writing. Those of you who worked your way through and managed the science in Part Two can thank her. As a non-scientist, she was insistent that it stay in the book.

I would like to recognize the many thousands of individuals who work silently and quietly in institutions and laboratories around the world. These often unrecognized people unravel the complexity of the human body and mind fragment by fragment, allowing us to hopefully one day remove the scourge of cancer and other terrible diseases from society. I may sometimes have critiques of the politics of the scientific world, but the individuals who work long hours for small financial rewards and recognition should be applauded. The many thousands of pages I read record their diligence and commitment. We all owe them a great big thank you.

My sister, Pelly, whose farm allowed me the space to finish this work. A haven from the chaotic world outside. More than that, her quiet wisdom and observations on human nature and that of animals guided some of my thinking.

Of course my family, my wife, Camille, who put up with me for years, and my children, Mat and Morgan, who often had to deal with being second place to my patients. Thank you for being such great friends today.

The team at Scribe: First, my editor, Jenny, who helped turn a lot of information in a terribly written manuscript into a book that is both readable and interesting. Without your skill, it would be languishing in a pile of poorly written books. I cannot thank you enough. Candace, who corrected my appallingly written English, and Caroline, who helped shape the layout, and Samantha who's sharp eyes put the finishing touches on the book. To Beth, who helped me come up with the correct title. To Becca and Erin, my publishing managers who directed the transition from scribbling to publication. Oceana, who designed the cover. I love it. And lastly, Tucker and his team, whose idea makes it possible for individuals to share their knowledge as authors under the direction of professionals.

My parents, who somehow managed to instill in me the firm belief that it was OK to be different. More importantly, that it was critical to think outside the box, to respectfully question everything and everyone, even those in authority and so-called experts. Both believed in equality of the sexes and the importance of both men and women in shaping a better world. Their own lives and careers speak for themselves.

Finally, you the reader for giving up your own precious time to read this book and take the risk that this time might be wasted. I can only hope that you are happy that you did so and in some way it has changed your life for the better.

ABOUT THE AUTHOR

Dr. Sam was born in Sheffield, England in 1961. His father was one of England's first industrial physicians, and his mother was a human physical therapist who introduced sports physical therapy into the world of equine sports and dog racing. Dr. Sam's formative years were spent on a small holding and eventually small farm, where he learned not only how to enjoy his own company but also the skills of farming. As so many "middle-class" English, he was sent away to boarding school; for him, as for others, it was a traumatic experience that shaped his entire life.

Always independent and a bit of a maverick, a legacy of his childhood, he charted his own career path, which was wildly interesting and chaotic, often stressful, but always growing. He survived his teenage years by diving into biology and ecology, which led to an understanding of cooperative systems. He weathered the emotional and physical challenges of this period by embracing Buddhist philosophy, and he would argue psychology at eighteen years of age. These two interests, ecology and Buddhism, have been the backbone upon which he built his life. His main curse and blessing is that his ever-inquiring mind forgot to stop asking, Why? He trained in medicine and surgery at St. Thomas' Hospital, London—a historic institution located across the River Thames from the Houses of Parliament and Big Ben. His passion for *why* has led him down several paths, but all are linked in some way to his fundamental belief that all things are connected and that success is based not so much upon survival of the fittest, but rather cooperative behaviors.

Not only has he had an interesting career in medicine working across a broad range of specialties and championing functional and holistic approaches to the care of patients, but he is also an experienced large and small boat sailor and pilot, flying many different aircraft, including jets and gliders. In addition to his medical degree, he holds master's degrees in aviation safety systems and human factors, and gastroenterology and nutrition. Dr. Sam, as he is known, is passionate about life in general and his work in particular, and this book shares his pragmatic common-sense approach to being healthy in this crazy, modern world. It is based on his own personal journey, those of his patients, and literally thousands of hours of reading and research. If you ask him how he has the time for all this, he'll smile and reply, "I don't watch television, and I sleep seven hours."